Health&Fitness
MAGAZINE

SHAPE UP AT HOME

Words Caroline Sandry
Cover photography Ian Derry
Photography Will Ireland
Models Willow @ MOT, Jacqueline Freeman @ MOT
Clothing Nike (www.nikestore.com); Brooks (www.brooksrunning.co.uk);
Casall (www.casallstore.com); Freddy (020 7836 5291); Asics (www.asics.co.uk);
adidas (www.adidas.com); American Apparel (www.americanapparel.net);
Puma (www.puma.com); No Balls (www.noballs.co.uk);
Shock Absorber (www.shockabsorber.co.uk).

Equipment Casall (www.casallstore.com), Reebok (www.reebokfitness.co.uk);
Physio Supplies (www.physiosupplies.com); Pro Fitness (www.pro-fitness.com).
Art editors Holly White, Victoria Hill
Design Louise Browne
Sub-editors Eve Boggenpoel, Emma Morris, Margaret Bartlett
Nutrition expert Angela Dowden
Editor Mary Comber
Editorial director Pete Muir

Digital production manager Nicky Baker
Bookazine manager Dharmesh Mistry
Production director Robin Ryan
Managing director of advertising Julian Lloyd-Evans
Newstrade director Martin Belson
Publishing director Richard Downey
Deputy managing director James Burnay
Chief operating officer Brett Reynolds
Group finance director Ian Leggett
Chief executive James Tye
Chairman Felix Dennis

MAG**BOOK**

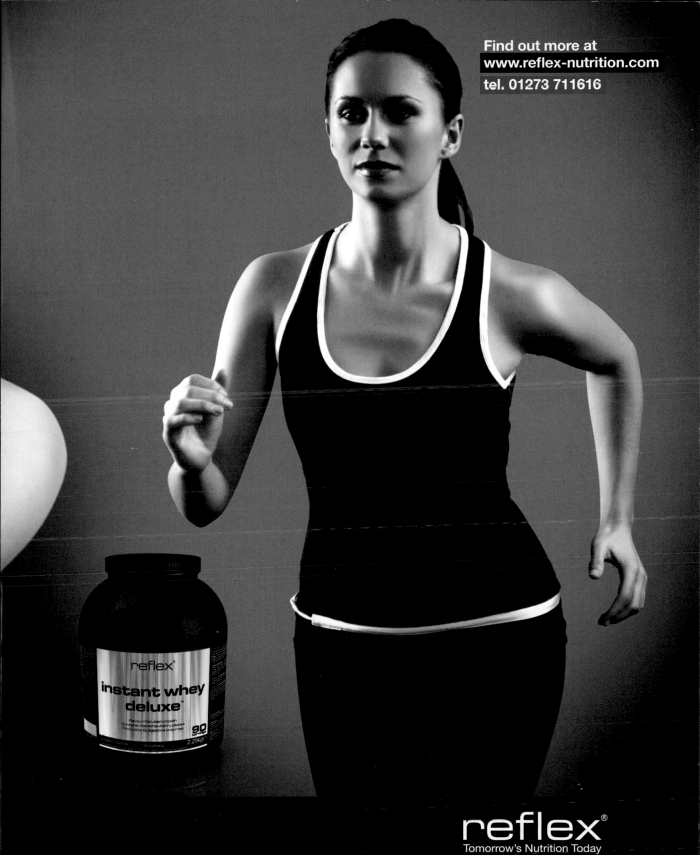

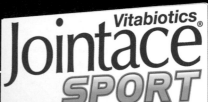
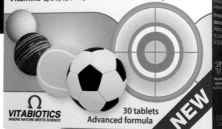

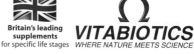

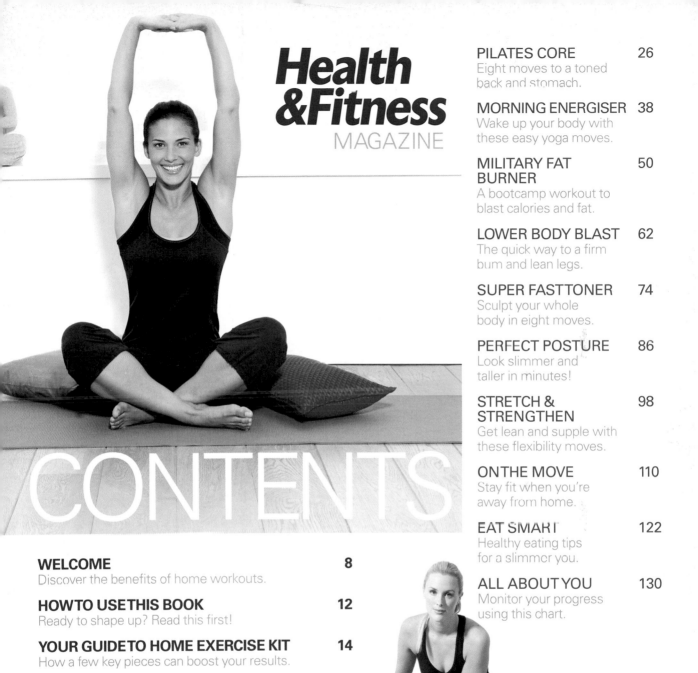

Health &Fitness
MAGAZINE

CONTENTS

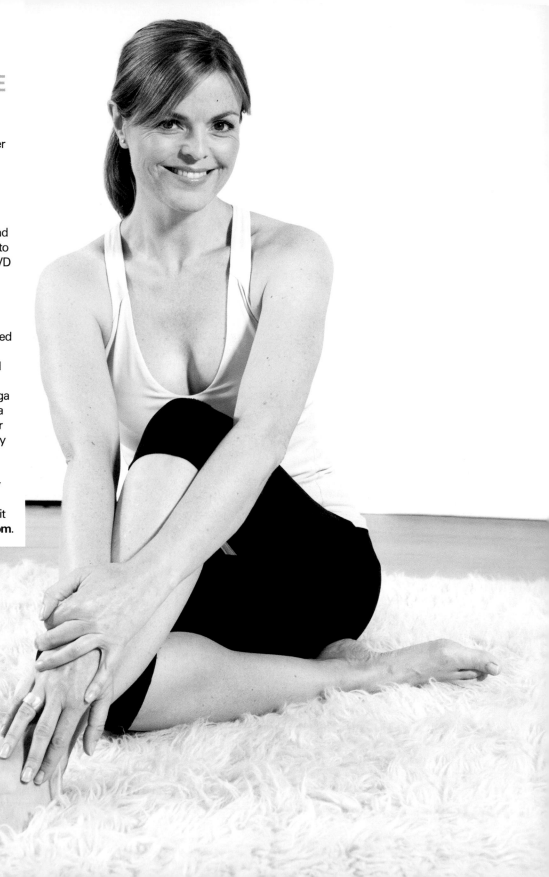

ABOUT THE
AUTHOR

Caroline Sandry is a Pilates and yoga teacher and a personal trainer. An established fitness presenter and writer, Caroline regularly appears on Body in Balance TV, QVC UK and has eight fitness DVDs to her name. Her latest DVD is *Pilates with Caroline Sandry* – three great Pilates workouts for a leaner body and flatter tum. Caroline has worked with many celebrities including actresses and models. 'By combining fitness training with yoga and Pilates, I can tailor a programme suitable for any fitness level or body shape. This book gives you the tools to do the same. I hope you enjoy it!' For more info, or to buy Caroline's DVD, visit **www.carolinesandry.com**.

WELCOME

You're probably reading this book because you want to shape up quickly and easily. Perhaps you've no time for the gym, want to save money or need inspiring exercise ideas to fit your lifestyle. The good news is, this guide offers a range of home workouts to suit all your goals. Whether you want to firm your bottom, improve your fitness or tone up all over, you'll find a quick and easy solution. *Shape up at Home* will help you sculpt your body, stretch and strengthen your muscles and de-stress your mind – without stepping outside the door.

Exercising at home can be just as effective as a gym workout – for a fraction of the time and effort. With just a few pieces of kit, you can achieve the same results you would at a health club. You can turn up at your own private gym (your lounge!) in your PJs, and if your mascara runs, who cares?

Variety is crucial to successful training, so this book has a range of exercise plans, from hard-core bootcamp circuits to energising yoga sequences. By following the exercises and nutrition tips, you can slim down, boost your health and fitness, strengthen your muscles, improve your posture and energy levels, and stay youthful and vibrant for life!

WHY EXERCISE AT HOME?

It saves time
With no travel time, you maximise your results per minute!

It's flexible
You can select a workout to suit your mood on the day. If you've planned a run, but wake up feeling groggy, you can simply roll out your mat and do some energising yoga moves instead.

You can exercise when it suits you
Whether you work shifts, are an early bird or want to split your exercise into two segments over the day – you choose when you work out.

It builds your confidence
If you find training in a gym intimidating, working out at home means you can build strength and learn new techniques.

It boosts your mood
Some of the cardiovascular exercise we'll recommend is outdoors. Training in the fresh air benefits your mind and body and can really lift your mood.

It's convenient
You don't have the hassle of packing your gym kit and toiletries, or travelling to and from the gym.

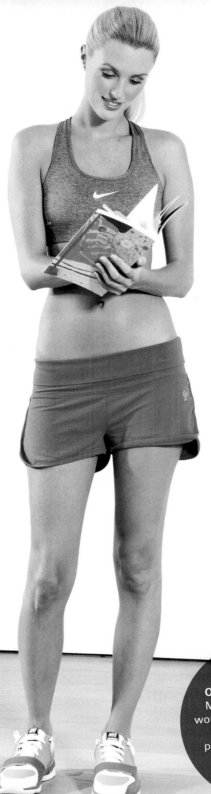

THE BENEFITS OF
USING THIS BOOK

Better posture
You'll strengthen the often-neglected muscles of the upper back to improve your shoulder alignment and function.

A flat stomach
Your deep core muscles will become stronger, flattening your stomach and improving your posture and spine health.

Toned legs and bum
The lower-body exercises will strengthen and shape your legs and bottom, particularly your gluteals, hamstrings and quadriceps.

Stronger heart and lungs
Your heart and lung strength will improve as a result of the interval-style training and additional cardiovascular exercise you do.

Better flexibility
The yoga and cool-down sequences will help lengthen your muscles and increase your flexibility.

Weight loss
By building lean muscle tissue, you'll boost your metabolism, helping you lose weight.

KEEP TRACK OF YOUR PROGRESS
Making notes on your workouts helps you create a balanced exercise programme. You'll also be able to track your improvements.

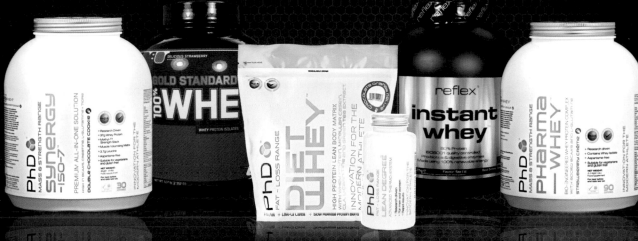
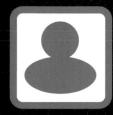 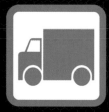 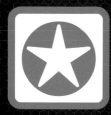 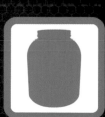

HOW TO USE

❶ SELECT YOUR ROUTINE

This plan is based around eight different workouts that vary in theme and intensity. You can select your workout according to your fitness goals and your mood. If you're feeling tired and stiff, go for Stretch & Strengthen or the Morning Energiser.

If your problem area is your lower body, do the Lower Body Blast twice a week, and select a further routine of your choice. Or, if you haven't done any cardiovascular exercise one week, go for the Military Fat Burner.

As a general rule, try to work out three to five times a week. All of these sessions work your body against resistance, and three of the plans train your cardiovascular system (see page 18 for ideas). Each workout has a step-by-step guide to ensure your technique is correct, and there's plenty of variety to keep your body challenged and ensure your workouts never get stale.

❷ PREPARE YOUR BODY

We've included a warm-up (page 22) to prepare your body for exercise and a cool-down (page 24) to stretch you out after your workout to help prevent injury. These should top and tail every exercise session.

❸ WORK YOUR HEART

As well as following the exercise plans, you should also train your heart and lungs with cardiovascular exercise, which will help burn calories and fat for weight loss. Turn to page 18 for more details.

❹ EAT SMART

As with any fitness or weight-loss plan, your diet plays a key role in helping you get in shape, so we've dedicated a chapter to nutritional advice to help you on your way. See page 122.

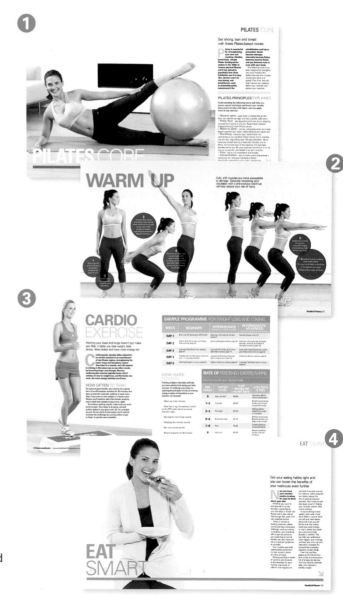

THIS BOOK

Ready to start? Read this first!

THE WORKOUTS

PILATES CORE PAGE 26

This is a strengthening routine that uses a mat and an exercise ball. It focuses mainly on your core muscles, although your entire body will reap the benefits.

MORNING ENERGISER PAGE 38

This invigorating routine is based on a yoga sun salutation and will stretch you from top to toe, waking your body and mind while getting you in great shape.

MILITARY FAT BURNER PAGE 50

Based on military training exercises, this plan is an intense and powerful workout for your entire body, including your heart and lungs.

LOWER BODY BLAST PAGE 62

Want to lift your bottom and sculpt your legs? These exercises will tone and strengthen your lower body.

SUPER-FAST TOTAL BODY TONER PAGE 74

The perfect 12-minute body blast, for when time is tight but you still need impressive results.

POSTURE PERFECT PAGE 86

Balance your body and strengthen the postural muscles of your shoulders and spine and you'll look instantly slimmer.

STRETCH & STRENGTHEN PAGE 98

Mobilise your joints and lengthen your muscles as you strengthen and tone. This routine is a relaxing and revitalising plan, leaving you feeling supple and flexible.

ON THE MOVE PAGE 110

Whether you're in a hotel on holiday or stuck at the office, this routine will shape and tone your whole body, using only your body weight and the furniture in your room!

WHAT YOU NEED TO GET STARTED

You don't need high-tech gear or a home gym to follow this book. These are your only essentials.

An exercise mat
A yoga or Pilates mat is ideal. You may find a Pilates mat is a little more cushioned.

Trainers
It's a good idea to invest in a decent pair of trainers. Take time to look for a proper sports store, as you may find you need a pair of corrective trainers if you've experienced any problems with your feet in the past.

Sports bra
When you exercise, even at home, your breasts move a surprising amount. This can be uncomfortable and may stretch the breast tissue, which can lead to a sagging bust. A proper sports bra will improve your comfort levels and posture, as well as your performance.

Water
Have some water handy, particularly if it's a hot day or you're planning a long session (more than 45 minutes).
For more kit ideas, see page 14.

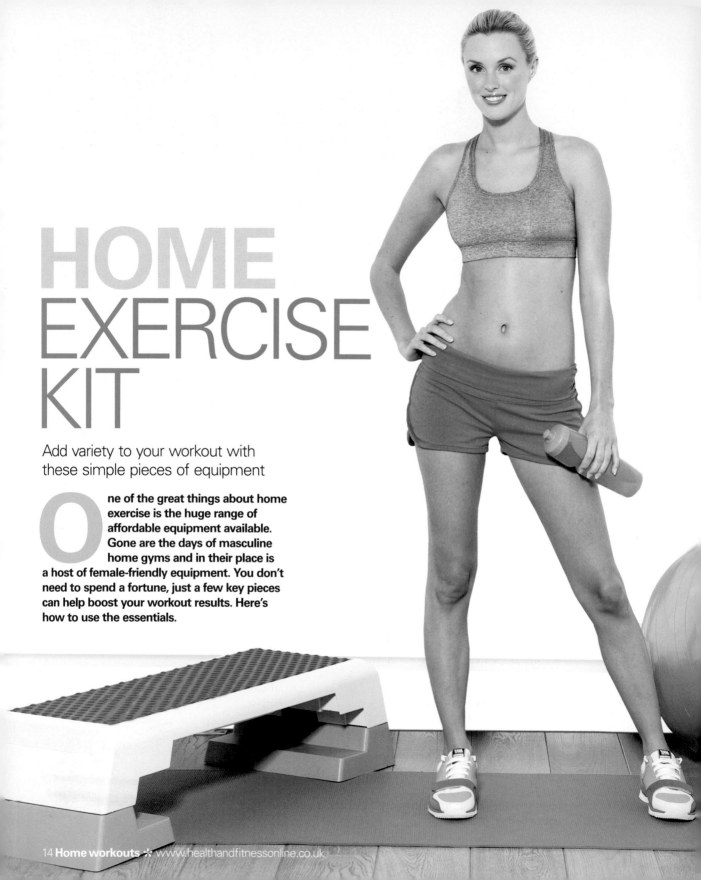

HOME EXERCISE KIT

Add variety to your workout with these simple pieces of equipment

One of the great things about home exercise is the huge range of affordable equipment available. Gone are the days of masculine home gyms and in their place is a host of female-friendly equipment. You don't need to spend a fortune, just a few key pieces can help boost your workout results. Here's how to use the essentials.

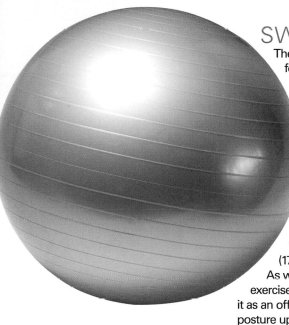

SWISS BALL

These air-filled balls are great for core-strength exercises. Performing your regular exercises while sitting or lying on the ball's unstable surface adds a challenge as your core muscles work to stabilise you. The balls come in three sizes – choose one according to your height: 55cm – up to 5'5" (165cm); 65cm – 5'6"–5'9"; (166–175cm); 75cm – 5'10" (177cm) upwards.

As well as using your ball for exercise, you can sit on it and use it as an office chair to help keep your posture upright and gently exercise your stability muscles while you work!

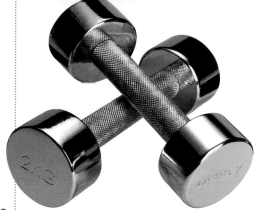

DUMBBELLS

Using dumbbells is the perfect way to sculpt your body. Unlike using weights at a gym, where your body is static (sitting on a bench with your back supported, for example), using dumbbells for resistance work means you engage your stabilising muscles to keep upright.

If your budget can stretch to it, select two different weights, so you can gradually progress and challenge different muscles. Alternatively, buy a stack of weights, ranging from 3–12kg, for a complete home gym that takes up the same space as two shoeboxes.

You'll know you're using the correct weight when you have exhausted the working muscle in the last repetition of a set of exercises. As a general guide for upper-body exercises, start with 3–5 kg. To add resistance to lower-body moves, such as squats, try 8–10 kg. And remember, muscle burns more calories than fat, so pick up those weights!

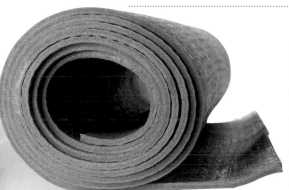

MAT

A decent mat is your first investment, as it will cushion your spine when doing exercises that involve lying on the floor. A mat will also provide a non-slip surface for yoga and Pilates moves and protect your carpet from all that sweat you'll be producing!

KETTLEBELLS

Looking like small cannon balls with a handle attached, these weights originate from Russia, first appearing in a Russian dictionary in 1704, and are still used by the Russian military.

Some kettlebells may look a little masculine and scary, but these weights give an incredible workout. Many of the exercises are based on a swinging movement, which makes you engage your core stabilising muscles to help control the momentum. You'll quickly feel your heart rate pick up, so it's a great form of cardiovascular training as well. On rainy days, you could do a kettlebell circuit instead of a run and boost your strength too.

Before using kettlebells at home, it's worth attending a class to learn good technique to avoid injury and muscle soreness. Start with a 6–8kg kettlebell.

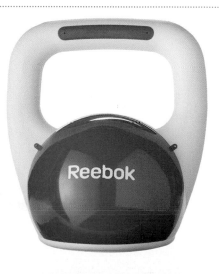

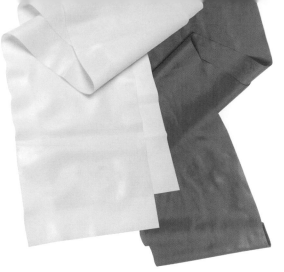

RESISTANCE BAND

This is perhaps the simplest piece of resistance kit there is! The stretchy band, made of elastic rubber or latex, weighs virtually nothing and can fold up in the palm of your hand – perfect if you live in a small flat or travel frequently.

The band can be used in place of weights to perform regular exercises, such as biceps curls and triceps extensions, as well as the moves shown in this guide.

Using a band builds muscle tone and strength and, because of its elasticity, your muscles will be challenged as they contract and lengthen. The closer you hold it to your moving limb, the stronger the resistance.

When holding the band, make a fist and keep your hands in line with your arms, not letting your wrists flex or bend. Always keep your shoulders away from your ears.

A medium-strength band is a good starting point, or you can use an exercise tube with handles if you prefer.

STAY SAFE

Avoid injury and make your workouts as enjoyable as possible, by following these safety points.

○ Always warm up and cool down (see pages 22 and 24).
○ Stay hydrated. It's best to be hydrated before you train, so aim to drink around 500ml of water, two to three hours before exercising, and another 250ml 15 minutes before you start.
○ Wear non-slip shoes or use a non-slip mat if you prefer to exercise barefoot.
○ Make sure you have enough space around you. This sounds obvious, but you don't want to swing your kettlebell into the TV!
○ Don't exercise if you're not feeling well.
○ Many of these exercises are not suitable during pregnancy.
○ Avoid training the same muscles with resistance on two consecutive days, as they need time to heal and repair.

MEDICINE BALL

A medicine ball is the size of a basketball, but usually weighs between 3–9kg. It can be used for traditional weight-lifting exercises, or you can use it explosively to create speed and power. For example, perform a sit-up with a partner and, as you lift your head and shoulders, explosively throw the ball from your chest to your partner. Your partner throws it back and you catch it as you lower your shoulders back to the floor with control.

For the exercises in this book, I recommend you use a 4kg ball.

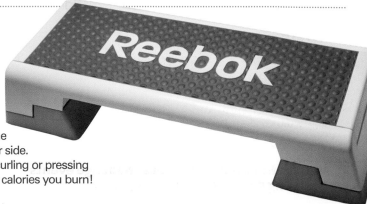

STEP

A Step is a great, low-cost piece of equipment for an effective cardio workout. Just keep moving for the recommended time and vary your steps. For example:
○ Step up and down.
○ Jog up and down.
○ Step sideways up and down.
○ Step up with left leg then pull your right knee up in the air in front of you. Step down and repeat on the other side.
○ Use your arms on any of the above moves – biceps curling or pressing arms out in front of you. The more you move the more calories you burn!

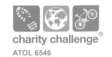

charity challenge®
ATOL 6546

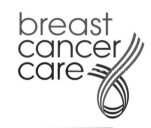

breast
cancer
care

Follow in the footsteps of
Denise Van Outen and Fearne Cotton
Trek Peru for Breast Cancer Care

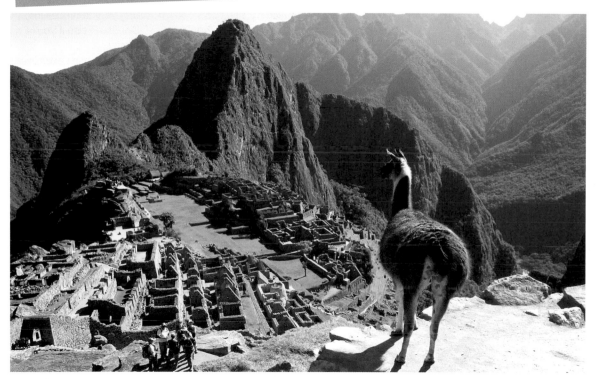

Denise and Fearne challenge you to take on this journey to Machu Picchu and raise money to support people affected by breast cancer

29 April – 8 May 2011
16 – 25 September 2011
13 – 22 April 2012

For more information or to register
visit www.breastcancercare.org.uk/events
call 0845 092 0805 quoting HFMAG

We also have other overseas challenge events including China, Kenya and the Sahara.

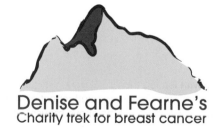

Denise and Fearne's
Charity trek for breast cancer

Registered charity in England & Wales 1017658 Registered charity in Scotland SC038104

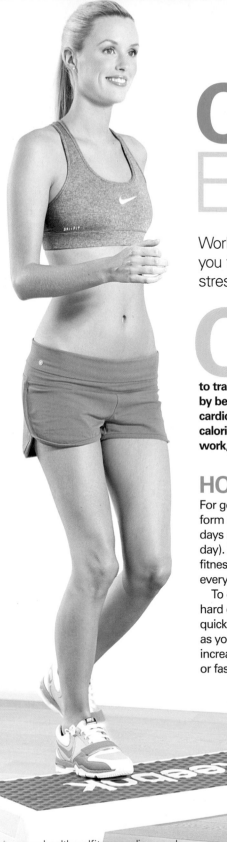

CARDIO EXERCISE

Working your heart and lungs doesn't just make you fitter, it helps you lose weight, beat stress, sleep better and have more energy too

Cardiovascular exercise (often referred to as aerobic exercise) is an essential part of any fitness regime, strengthening the heart, lungs and circulatory system. Your heart is a muscle and will respond to training in the same way as any other muscle, by becoming larger and stronger. Because cardiovascular exercise typically burns a lot of calories, it's key to weight loss, and the harder you work, the more energy (calories) you'll burn.

HOW OFTEN TO TRAIN

For general good health you need to do a gentle form of cardiovascular exercise for 30 minutes, five days a week (for example, walking to work every day). If you want to lose weight or enhance your fitness, you'll need to add a few harder sessions every week (see sample programme, right).

To continue getting results, make sure you work hard enough. Your body is amazing, and will quickly adapt to any given task. So, for example, as your 3k run starts to feel easier, you'll need to increase the challenge by running either longer or faster to get the same benefits.

SAMPLE PROGRAMME FOR WEIGHT LOSS AND TONING

WEEK	BEGINNER	INTERMEDIATE (Exercising for at least six months)	INTERMEDIATE/ADVANCED (Exercising regularly for at least a year)
DAY 1	Brisk walk 25–30 minutes, RPE level 6	Step, jog or fast walk 45 minutes, level 6–7	Run 40 minutes, level 7–8
DAY 2	Walk or Step 20 minutes, plus Pilates Core workout, page 36	Morning Energiser workout, page 48	Interval run (3 minutes fast, 3 minutes recovery), level 6–9, plus Stretch & Strengthen workout, page 108
DAY 3	Super-fast Total Body Toner workout, page 84	Fast walk 20 minutes, plus Lower Body Blast workout, page 72	Brisk walk or Step 20 minutes, level 6, plus Pilates Core workout, page 36
DAY 4	Walk/jog intervals 25 minutes (3 minutes walk, 1 minute jog), level 6–7	Jog intervals 30 minutes (2 minutes fast, 3 minutes slow), level 7–8	Military Fat Burner workout, page 60
DAY 5	Morning Energiser workout, page 48	Military Fat Burner workout, page 60	Super-fast Total Body Toner workout, page 84

HOW HARD TO WORK

Training at higher intensities will help you burn calories both during and after exercise. To challenge your body, try applying the principles of interval training (using a variety of intensities) to your exercise. For example:

○ Warm up, three minutes.

○ Walk fast or jog, five minutes, level 6 on the RPE scale (rate of perceived exertion), right.

○ Run fast for one minute, level 8.

○ Walk/jog, five minutes, level 6.

○ Run one minute, level 8.

○ Repeat sequence for 30 minutes.

As your fitness improves, gradually build up to three to five minutes of effort and three to five minutes at recovery pace.

RATE OF PERCEIVED EXERTION (RPE)

How to monitor your training levels

RPE SCALE	EFFORT LEVEL	% OF MAXIMUM HEART RATE	HOW DOES IT FEEL
0	Very, very light	40–50	Very easy, able to hold a conversation.
1–2	Very light	50–60	Breathing somewhat harder, but still able to converse easily.
3–4	Fairly light	60–65	Feeling slightly breathless, harder to converse.
5–6	Somewhat hard	65–75	Difficult to converse. Breathing faster and beginning to sweat.
7–8	Hard	75–85	Breathing heavily, sweating heavily.
9	Very hard	85–95	Breathing difficult, hard to maintain the level.
10	Very, very hard	95–100	Unable to continue for long, may feel nauseous.

BE YOUR OWN PERSONAL TRAINER

Get more from your workouts with these expert training secrets

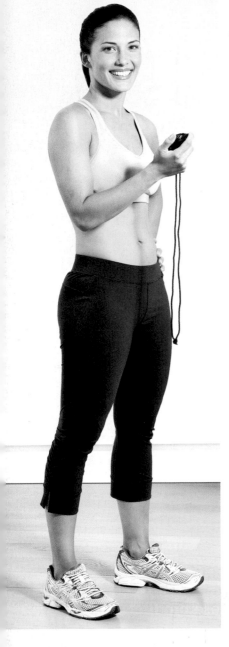

So you have the kit, the exercises and are raring to go. To get the best results from your sessions, follow these top personal trainer tips, and coach yourself to success.

SET GOALS

○ A personal trainer's first job is to establish your starting point and your fitness and weight-loss goals. So grab some paper and a pen. Now write down today's date and your measurements – bust, waist, top hip (bony part), lower hip (often the widest part), thigh and upper arm. Be specific (for example, measure your thigh 22cm above your kneecap), so you hit the same spot each time.

○ You can weigh yourself if you prefer, but try not to get on the scales too frequently.

○ Now spend a few minutes thinking about a goal. Make this achievable in the near future (for example, I want to drop a dress size in eight weeks, or I want to be able to jog for 20 minutes non-stop).

○ Check your weight and measurements every two to four weeks to give your body the time to make changes, and record your progress in your notepad.

PROGRESS

Your body quickly adapts to challenges, so to avoid plateauing, increase the intensity or duration of your workouts every six to eight weeks. This could be using a heavier weight for an exercise, adding repetitions or increasing the length of time you exercise. For cardio work, such as jogging, only make 10 per cent increases in effort at a time to avoid injury.

GET MOTIVATED

Hopefully, you look forward to doing your workout, but we all hit times when our enthusiasm dwindles. Try these expert tips to stay on track.

○ Stick a photo on the fridge of someone you admire to remind you why you're on this journey.

○ Reward yourself. Arrange a nice meal out with a friend when you've completed your first month of training.

○ Give yourself pamper points! When you've reached a goal, treat yourself to a pamper session, such as a massage, to ease your achy but well-toned muscles!

○ Do it for charity – sign up for a charity event, such as a run, cycle, climb or hike.

PERFECT YOUR TECHNIQUE

Good technique is hugely important as it can help prevent injury. By using correct alignment during exercises (for example, keeping your shoulders back and down), you'll ensure the exercise hits the muscles intended.

○ Follow the step-by-step instructions in this book closely to ensure good form. If possible, use a mirror to check your alignment.

○ Always move through each exercise slowly and with control.

○ Aim to keep the muscles of your core engaged throughout each move.

○ If an exercise feels too hard, reduce the effort or rest a while.

○ If it feels too easy, increase the effort, weight or duration.

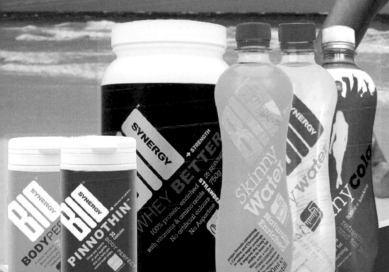

BIO SYNERGY
Make it Happen!

GET BEACH READY THIS
SUMMER
WITH OUR AWARD WINNING PRODUCTS
& 10 MINUTE TONE UP

Available online and at all good leading retailers including:

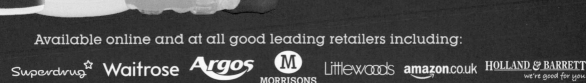

TESCO · *Superdrug* · Waitrose · **Argos** · **M** MORRISONS · Littlewoods · amazon.co.uk · HOLLAND & BARRETT *we're good for you*

For more information and real life success stories on these products, visit:
www.bio-synergy.co.uk or www.skinnywater.co.uk
OR CALL 020 7569 2528 TO RECEIVE YOUR FREE INFORMATION PACK, QUOTING PROMOTIONAL CODE TTU1

WARM UP

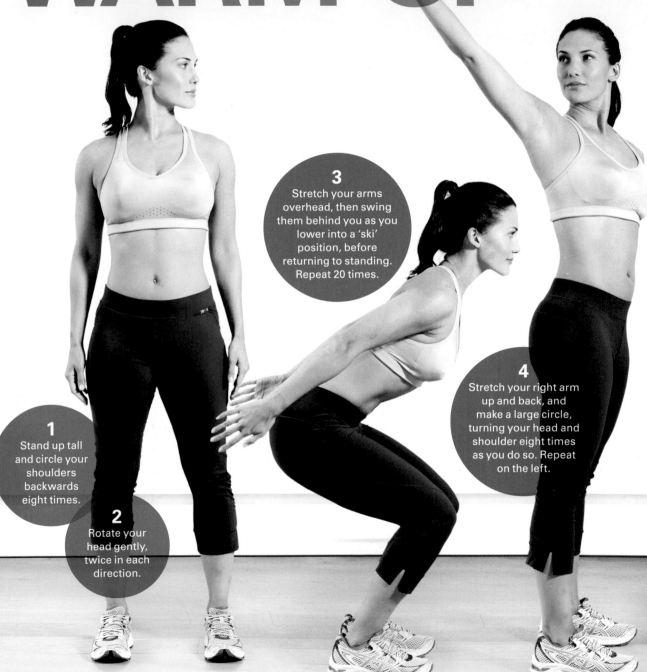

3
Stretch your arms overhead, then swing them behind you as you lower into a 'ski' position, before returning to standing. Repeat 20 times.

1
Stand up tall and circle your shoulders backwards eight times.

2
Rotate your head gently, twice in each direction.

4
Stretch your right arm up and back, and make a large circle, turning your head and shoulder eight times as you do so. Repeat on the left.

Cold, stiff muscles are more susceptible to damage. Gradually increasing your circulation with a pre-workout warm-up will help reduce your risk of injury

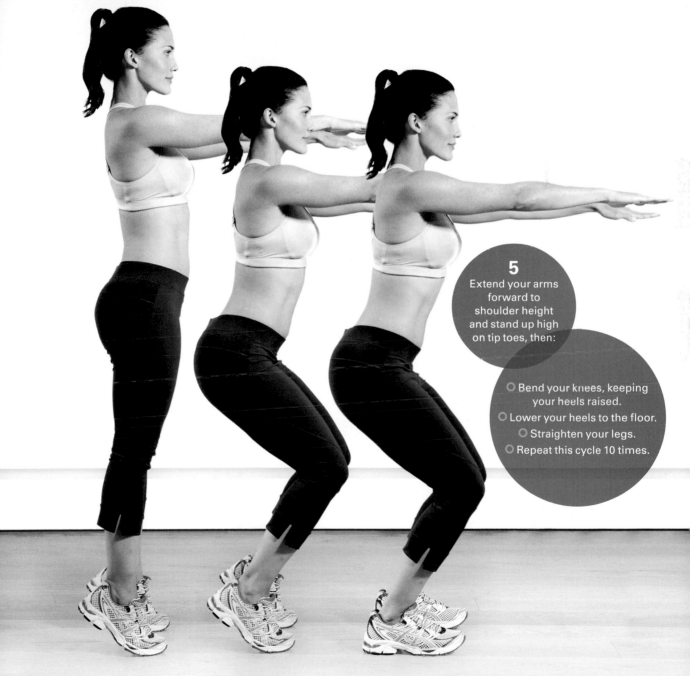

5
Extend your arms forward to shoulder height and stand up high on tip toes, then:

○ Bend your knees, keeping your heels raised.
○ Lower your heels to the floor.
○ Straighten your legs.
○ Repeat this cycle 10 times.

COOL DOWN

A cool-down session at the end of your routine helps flush waste products, such as lactic acid, from your muscles and minimises post-exercise muscle soreness

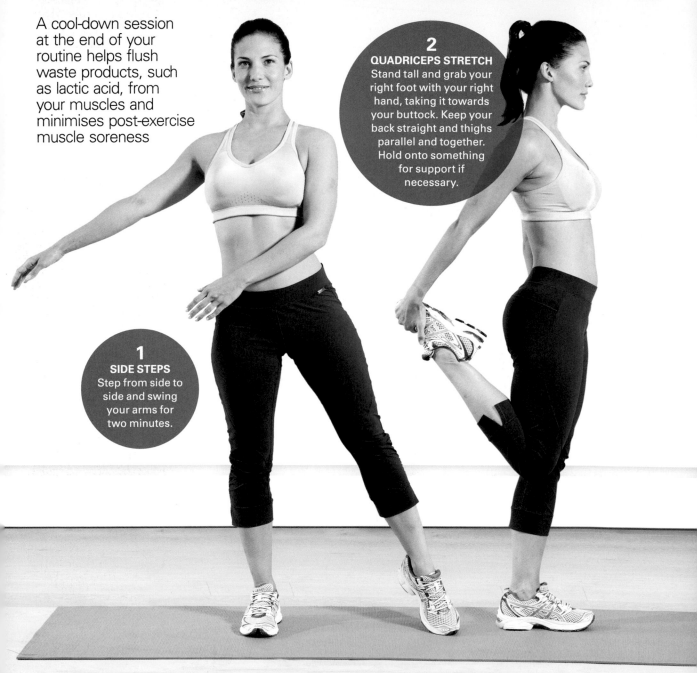

2
QUADRICEPS STRETCH
Stand tall and grab your right foot with your right hand, taking it towards your buttock. Keep your back straight and thighs parallel and together. Hold onto something for support if necessary.

1
SIDE STEPS
Step from side to side and swing your arms for two minutes.

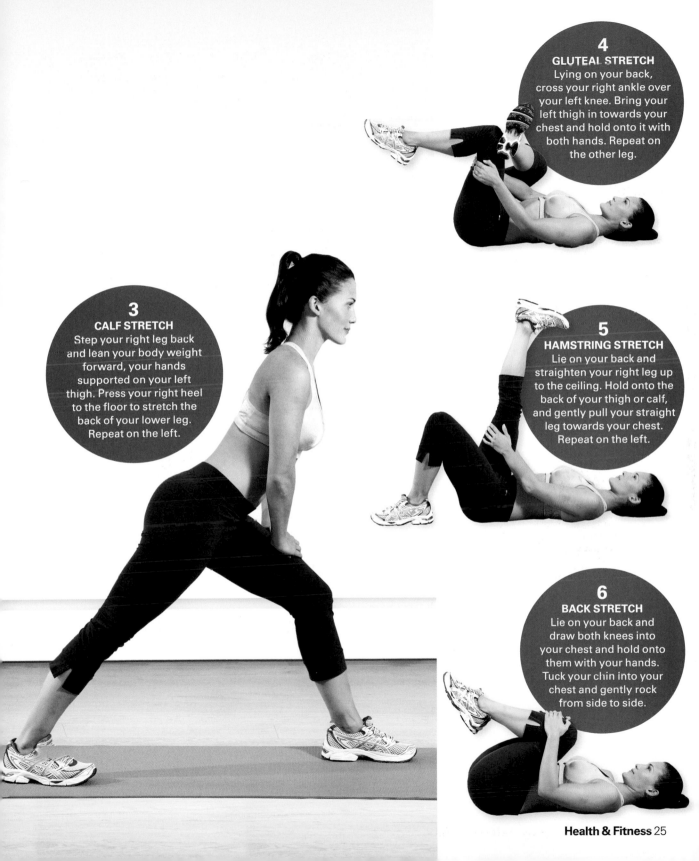

4
GLUTEAL STRETCH
Lying on your back, cross your right ankle over your left knee. Bring your left thigh in towards your chest and hold onto it with both hands. Repeat on the other leg.

3
CALF STRETCH
Step your right leg back and lean your body weight forward, your hands supported on your left thigh. Press your right heel to the floor to stretch the back of your lower leg. Repeat on the left.

5
HAMSTRING STRETCH
Lie on your back and straighten your right leg up to the ceiling. Hold onto the back of your thigh or calf, and gently pull your straight leg towards your chest. Repeat on the left.

6
BACK STRETCH
Lie on your back and draw both knees into your chest and hold onto them with your hands. Tuck your chin into your chest and gently rock from side to side.

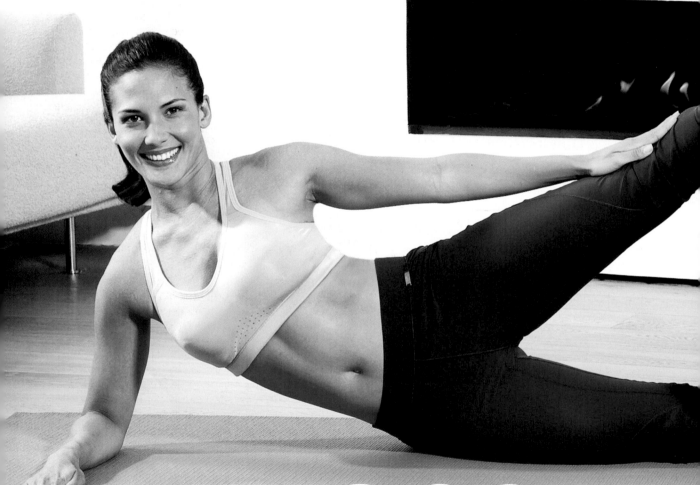

PILATES CORE

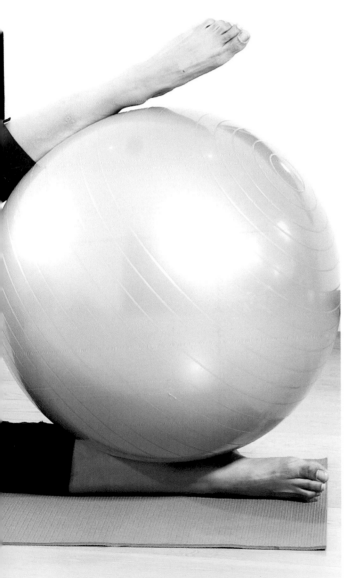

Get strong, lean and toned with these Pilates-based moves

Pilates is wonderful for strengthening your core and creating a flexible, toned body. Joseph Pilates developed the system in the 1920s to 'restore physical fitness', and it has gained in popularity ever since. Celebrities use it to stay slim, dancers use it to stay strong, and practitioners, such as physiotherapists, recommend it for rehabilitation and injury prevention. Backs become stronger, stomachs become flatter, bottoms become firmer and you become more in tune with your body.

The following routine has been designed to strengthen your core muscles (the abdominals and the muscles around your spine and pelvis). Over time, this will help improve your posture, flatten your stomach and reduce your waistline.

PILATES TERMS EXPLAINED

Understanding the following terms will help you ensure correct technique and boost your results. Once you're familiar with them, you can apply them to any exercise.

o **Neutral spine** – your back is neither flat on the floor, nor arched up high, but has a gentle, soft curve.
o **Pelvic floor** – the muscles you'd use to try stopping yourself from going to the loo. Keep these muscles engaged through each Pilates move.
o **Navel to spine** – exhale, and gently draw your belly button towards your spine, while keeping your spine still.
o **Breathing** – because your abdominals are contracted as you perform these moves, try to breathe into the ribs, expanding your ribcage outwards. Never hold your breath during an exercise. Breathe out on effort, the hardest part of the exercise. For example, breathe out as you lift your head and shoulders in an ab curl, or as you lift a dumbbell in an arm exercise.
o **Flow** – try to link movement and breath.
o **Concentration** – aim to make every movement a conscious act, and you'll develop a better mind-body connection and greater awareness. Use slow, controlled movements.

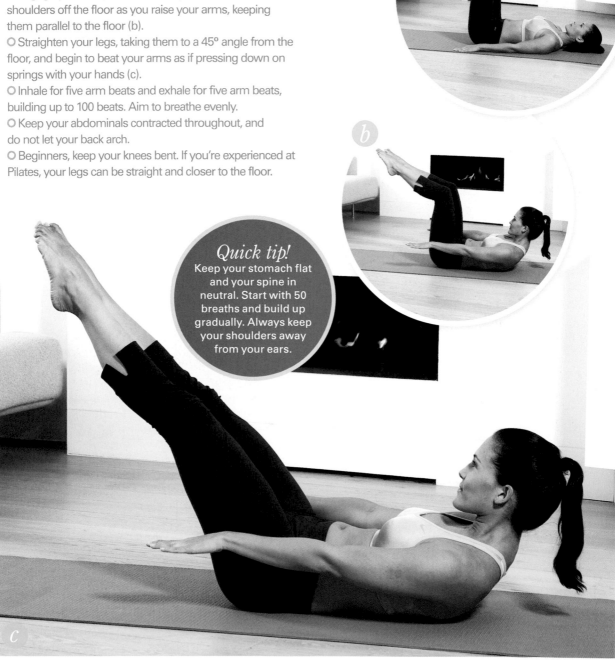

PILATES 100

BENEFITS: A fabulous core exercise that flattens your abdominals and strengthens your hip flexors.

○ Lie on your back, contract your abdominals and bring both knees up to a right angle with your thighs vertical (a).

○ Engage your core, exhale and lift your head and shoulders off the floor as you raise your arms, keeping them parallel to the floor (b).

○ Straighten your legs, taking them to a 45° angle from the floor, and begin to beat your arms as if pressing down on springs with your hands (c).

○ Inhale for five arm beats and exhale for five arm beats, building up to 100 beats. Aim to breathe evenly.

○ Keep your abdominals contracted throughout, and do not let your back arch.

○ Beginners, keep your knees bent. If you're experienced at Pilates, your legs can be straight and closer to the floor.

Quick tip!
Keep your stomach flat and your spine in neutral. Start with 50 breaths and build up gradually. Always keep your shoulders away from your ears.

PILATES CORE WORKOUT MOVES

ROLL-UP

BENEFITS: Mobilises your spine and strengthens your abdominals and core.

⚬ Sit up tall with your knees bent at 90° and your feet flat on the floor.

⚬ Hold your arms out in front of you at shoulder height, palms down and shoulders drawn away from your ears (a).

⚬ Draw your navel to your spine, engage your core and exhale as you tilt your pelvis, rolling – one vertebra at a time – half-way back towards the floor (b).

⚬ Inhale and roll back up, keeping your spine bent in a 'C' shape and your abdominals drawn inwards.

As you become stronger, straighten your legs and roll all the way to the floor without your feet lifting or legs tensing (c).

⚬ Repeat five to eight times.

Quick tip!
Keep navel to spine and your shoulders away from your ears.

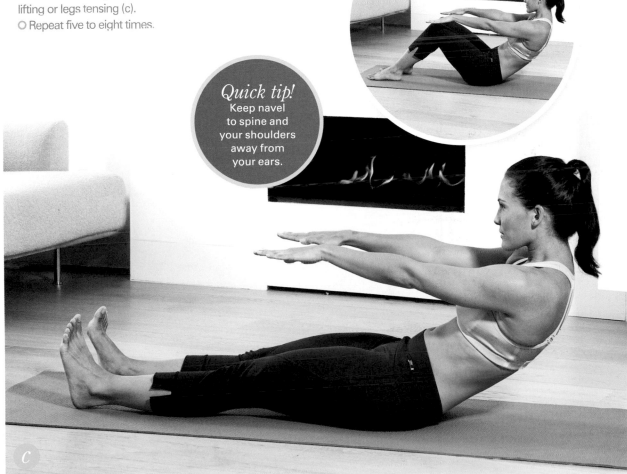

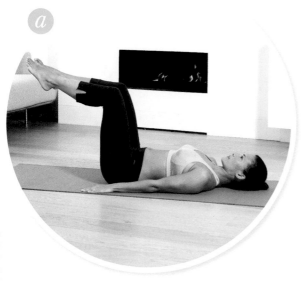

a

CRISS-CROSS

BENEFITS: Works your stomach, waist and thighs.

○ Lie on your back and bring your knees above your hips, knees bent at a right angle (a).
○ Place your fingertips behind your ears, keep your elbows wide and raise your head from the floor.
○ Exhale, and take your right shoulder to your left hip as you extend your right leg as low as you can. Aim to keep your stomach flat and your spine in neutral throughout (b).
○ Inhale, raise your right leg and return to centre.
○ Exhale, and repeat with the left shoulder travelling to the right hip, left leg extended.
○ Do 10 slow repetitions followed by 10 fast but controlled repetitions.

Quick tip!
Try to keep your stomach flat throughout, and move in a controlled manner. Don't let your hips rock as you move.

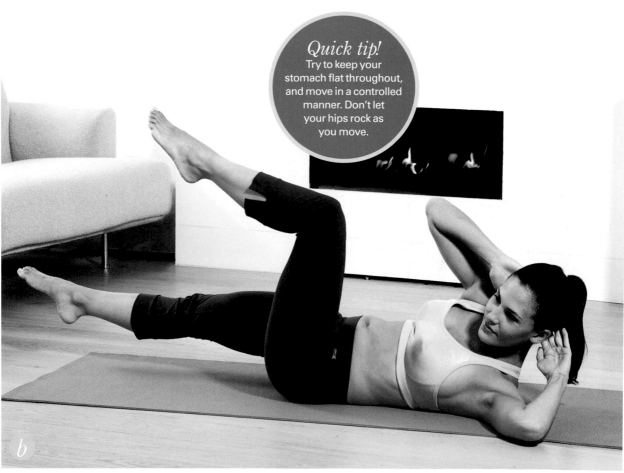

b

PILATES CORE WORKOUT MOVES

DART

BENEFITS: Strengthens your upper back and shoulders.

○ Lie on your front, hands by your sides, legs together, forehead resting on the floor.

○ Inhale, engage your pelvic floor and draw your shoulders away from your ears (a).

○ Exhale and lift your head and shoulders from the floor, reaching your hands towards your toes, thumbs facing the floor (b) and looking down at the mat.

○ Inhale and hold.

○ Exhale to return to the floor.

○ Do five to eight reps.

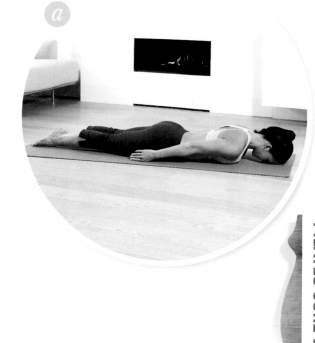

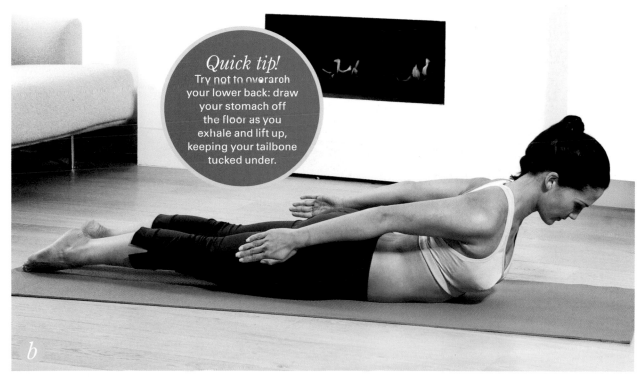

Quick tip!
Try not to overarch your lower back: draw your stomach off the floor as you exhale and lift up, keeping your tailbone tucked under.

PILATES CORE WORKOUT MOVES

PILATES CORE WORKOUT MOVES

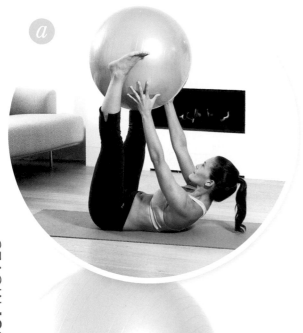

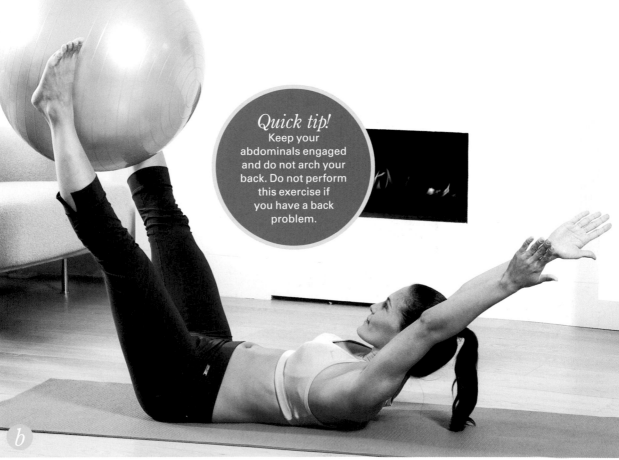

BALL PASS

BENEFITS: Targets the entire abdominal area, hip flexors, inner thighs, shoulders and chest.

○ Lie on your back with a Swiss ball between your calves.

○ Engage your abdominals and raise the ball until your feet are above your hips.

○ Flex your shoulders off the floor and reach up to take the ball into your hands (a).

○ Holding the ball, extend your arms back, making a 'V' shape between your hands and feet.

○ Bring your hands and feet back together, and pass the ball back between your calves.

○ Lower your legs slightly and extend your arms back, again forming a 'V' shape (b).

○ Continue passing the ball between your upper and lower body, building up to 10 reps.

Quick tip!
Keep your abdominals engaged and do not arch your back. Do not perform this exercise if you have a back problem.

SIDE BEND

BENEFITS: Strengthens your core, particularly your waist, and strengthens and tones shoulders and arms.

○ Sit on your left hip with your left knee bent in front of you. Your right knee should be raised, bent at 90°, and your right foot flat on the floor in front of your left foot. Rest your right hand on your raised knee, palm facing upwards.

○ Your left leg rests on the floor with your left foot just behind your right foot, and your body supported by your left arm.

○ Inhale to prepare and lengthen your supporting arm, drawing your torso away from the floor and your shoulders away from your ears (a).

○ Exhale, and lift your hips upwards (imagine your hips are being lifted in a sling), squeezing your inner thighs together and reaching your top arm over your head (b).

○ Inhale to bend your knees and return your hip back to the floor, hand back to your knee.

○ Repeat three to five times on each side.

○ To increase the intensity, hold a toning ball in the top hand.

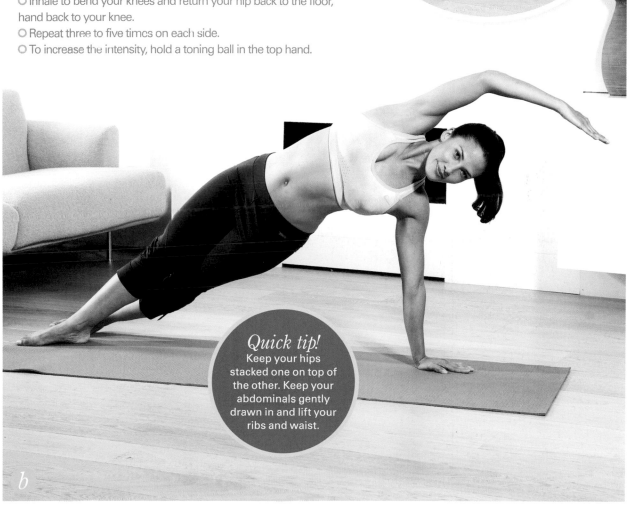

a

b

Quick tip!
Keep your hips stacked one on top of the other. Keep your abdominals gently drawn in and lift your ribs and waist.

SCISSORS

BENEFITS: Strengthens your core and legs.

○ Lie on your back, knees bent and hip-width apart, feet flat on the floor.

○ Exhale and draw your navel to your spine as you lift one leg at a time until your knees are above your hips and bent to a 90° angle. Inhale and raise your head and shoulders to look towards your knees.

○ Exhale as you straighten both legs and reach both hands around your left knee (a).

○ Inhale and lower your right leg towards the floor, bringing your left leg close to your face.

○ Exhale and pulse the lower leg twice, puffing out once on each pulse, as if blowing out candles.

○ Inhale as you switch legs by reaching the lower leg to the ceiling, and the upper leg to the floor, so they pass each other. Transfer your hands to hold the knee of the raised right leg (b).

○ Exhale as the second leg lowers and pulses twice. Continue with a smooth flowing motion, scissoring the legs apart. Repeat 16 times.

○ To increase the challenge, try performing this move with your arms by your sides, palms down and 15cm off the floor.

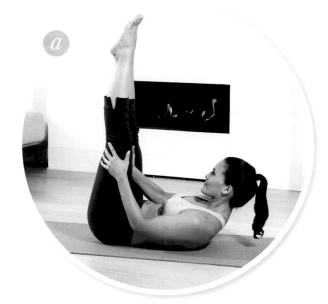

a

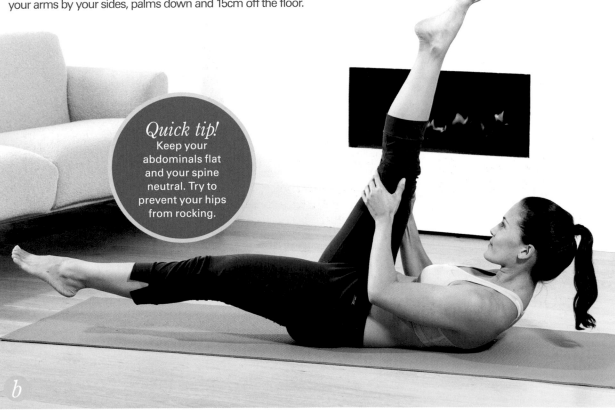

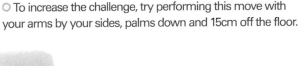

Quick tip!
Keep your abdominals flat and your spine neutral. Try to prevent your hips from rocking.

b

MERMAID

BENEFITS: Stretches out your waist and trunk.

○ Sit up tall on your left hip, with your feet out to the right, holding your right ankle with your right hand.

○ Reach your left arm to the ceiling, and inhale to stretch up (a).

○ Exhale to stretch over to your right, extending the left side of your ribs (b).

○ Repeat three times and then switch legs to repeat on the other side.

Quick tip!
Expand the area between your ribs and hips before flexing to the side. Always think of lengthening when you move.

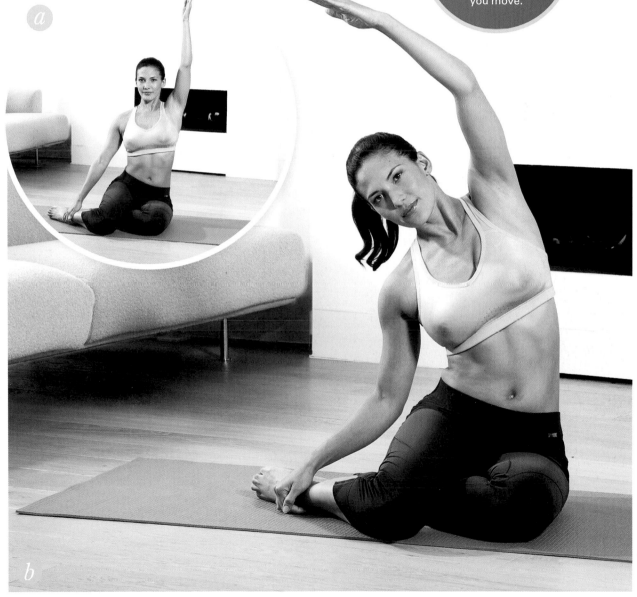

PILATES CORE WORKOUT MOVES

PILATES CORE CIRCUIT

Do these exercises two to three times a week. Apply the principles on page 27 to ensure correct technique and help you keep focused.

1 PILATES 100
REPS: UPTO 100
PAGE 28

2 ROLL-UP
REPS: 5–8
PAGE 29

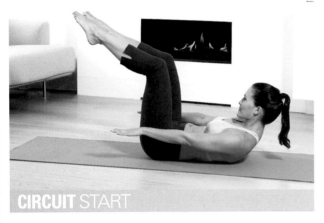

CIRCUIT START

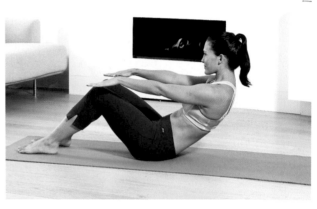

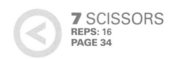

8 MERMAID
REPS: 3 EACH SIDE
PAGE 35

7 SCISSORS
REPS: 16
PAGE 34

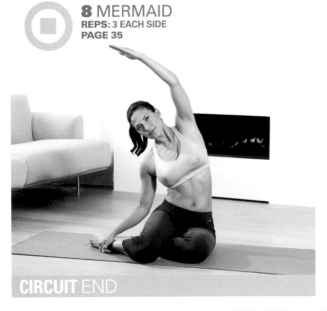

CIRCUIT END

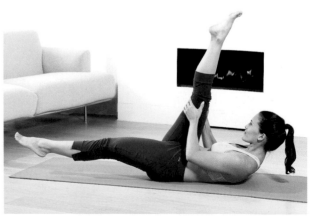

3 CRISS-CROSS
REPS: 10 SLOW, 10 FAST
PAGE 30

4 DART
REPS: 5–8
PAGE 31

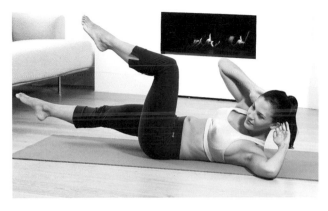

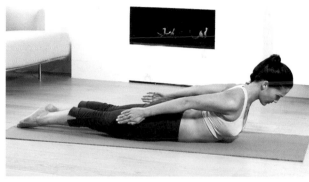

6 SIDE BEND
REPS: 3– 5 ON EACH SIDE
PAGE 33

5 BALL PASS
REPS: UP TO 10
PAGE 32

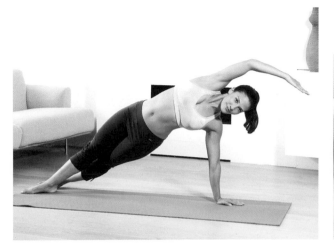

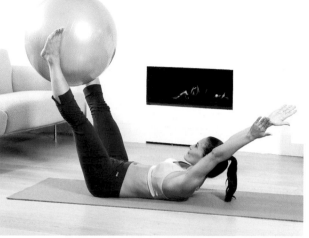

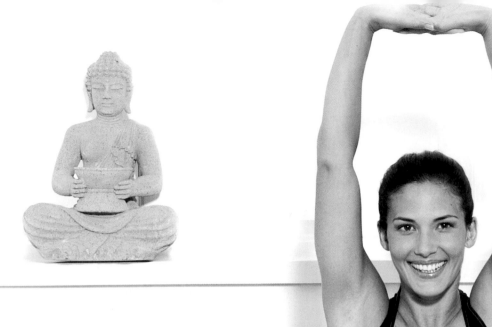

MORNING
ENERGISER

Wake up your body and mind with this yoga-based sequence designed to tone, stretch and strengthen

Mornings are a great time to exercise, and can really set you up for a healthy and energised day ahead. The following yoga-based moves will stretch out your entire body, leaving you refreshed, revitalised and ready for anything.

Many of us are so time-pressed, an extra half hour under the duvet may seem more appealing than an exercise session. But you'll feel really pleased with yourself if you make the effort – you'll be more alert, more supple and have much more energy to see you through the day. By stretching and challenging your entire body, you'll soon feel a lot fitter and stronger too.

A great tip is to get your clothes and kit ready the night before so there are no excuses when the alarm goes off! A flask of hot water with fresh lemon by your bed, prepared the night before, will be at the perfect drinking temperature for a refreshing drink to awaken your senses.

This sequence is based on the yoga sun salutation – traditionally performed towards the rising sun. Even if you don't get to see the sun, the rhythmic stretches gently ease your body from slumber to wakefulness. These moves strengthen and mobilise your spine, strengthen and tone your arms and core, and develop strength and balance in your lower body.

This routine is best performed on an empty stomach. If you do need to eat something first, try to keep it light, perhaps a piece of fruit or a small slice of granary toast, then wait at least 45 minutes before you start the sequence – this would be the ideal time for a wake-up walk around the block while your food digests!

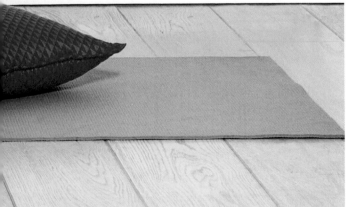

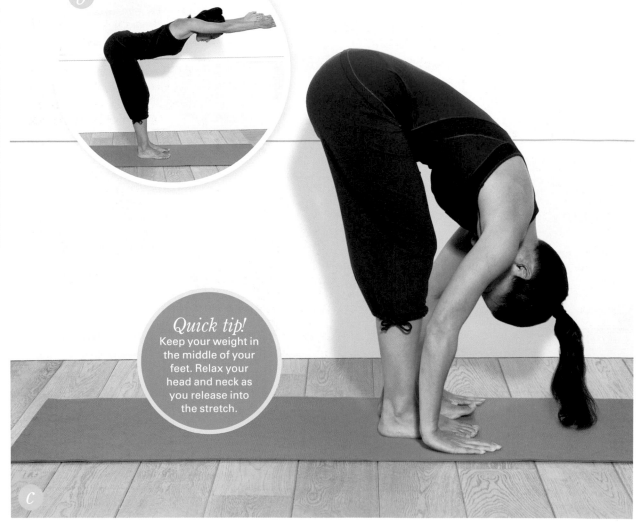

STANDING FORWARD BEND

BENEFITS: Stretches the entire back of your body.

○ Stand up tall, feet and knees together, arms by your sides.

○ Inhale and stretch your arms overhead, palms facing each other, upper arms by your ears (a).

○ Exhale and fold forward from your hips, keeping your spine straight (b), until your hands rest on the floor (c). Bend your knees if your hamstrings are tight.

○ Inhale and lift your head, shoulders and arms to flatten your spine (b).

○ Exhale and fold forward again (c).

○ Step your right foot back ready for lunge warrior.

Quick tip!
Keep your weight in the middle of your feet. Relax your head and neck as you release into the stretch.

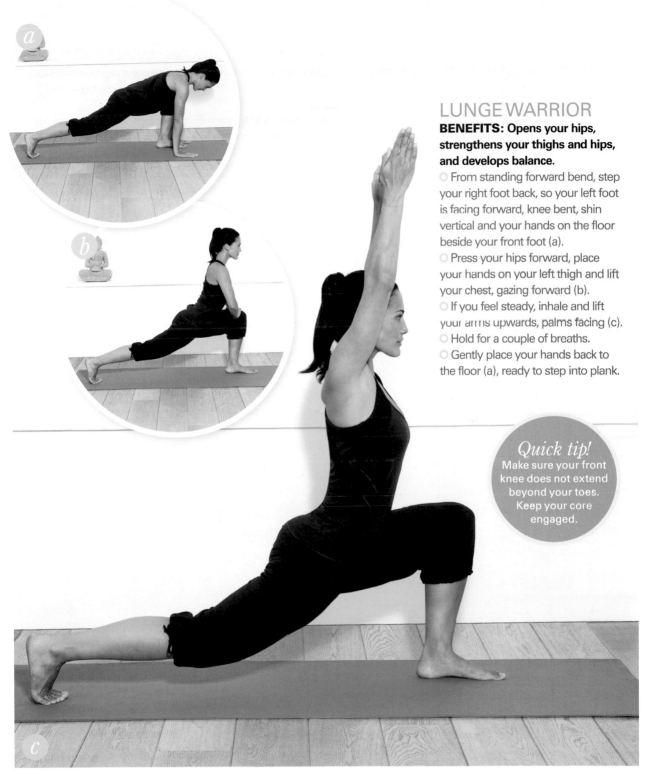

LUNGE WARRIOR

BENEFITS: Opens your hips, strengthens your thighs and hips, and develops balance.

○ From standing forward bend, step your right foot back, so your left foot is facing forward, knee bent, shin vertical and your hands on the floor beside your front foot (a).

○ Press your hips forward, place your hands on your left thigh and lift your chest, gazing forward (b).

○ If you feel steady, inhale and lift your arms upwards, palms facing (c).

○ Hold for a couple of breaths.

○ Gently place your hands back to the floor (a), ready to step into plank.

Quick tip!
Make sure your front knee does not extend beyond your toes. Keep your core engaged.

MORNING ENERGISER MOVES

MORNING ENERGISER MOVES

PLANK

BENEFITS: Originally a yoga move, the plank is renowned as a top core strengthener, working the deep abdominals, obliques, shoulders, back and pelvis.

○ From lunge warrior, step your left foot back to join your right, tightening your abdominals as you lift both knees off of the floor.

○ Keep your body in a straight line, spine in neutral and hands under your shoulders, fingers facing forward (pictured).

○ Hold for a couple of breaths, before moving into the crocodile.

Quick tip!
Keep your spine in neutral and your shoulders away from your ears. If you have back problems, keep one or both knees on the floor.

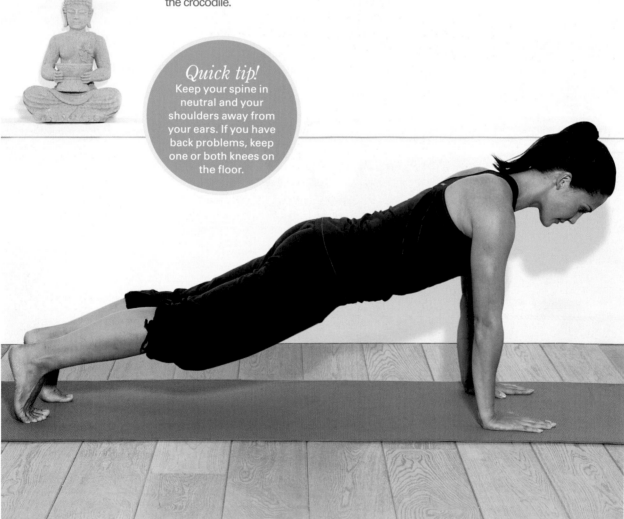

CROCODILE

BENEFITS: A top move for toned arms and core, this will give you definition in your shoulders and triceps.

○ From the plank position, keep your body in a straight line, bend your elbows keeping them close to your sides, and lower yourself towards the floor.

○ Try to hold your body above the floor in a straight line for one breath (pictured), before lowering to the floor, ready for cobra.

ADVANCED: For super strong arms and core, try a continuous circle of downward-facing dog (page 45) to plank to crocodile to dog, for a minute or more.

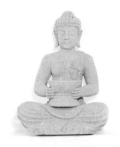

Quick tip!
Keep your abdominals drawn in tightly. If your arms are not yet strong enough, place your knees on the floor.

MORNING ENERGISER MOVES

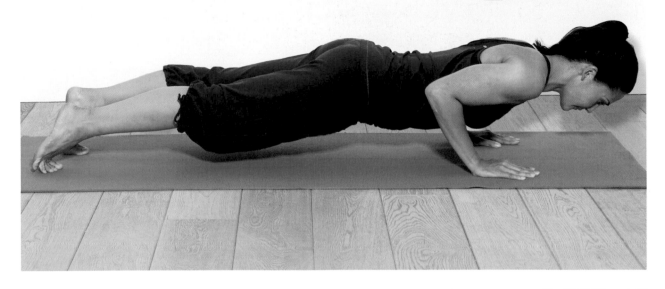

COBRA

BENEFITS: Mobilises your spine, strengthens your shoulders and spinal muscles. Counters rounded shoulders.

○ Lying face down, legs together and forehead on the floor, place your hands directly beneath your shoulders, palms down, fingers facing forwards.

○ Inhale and slowly raise your forehead, nose and then chin from the floor.

○ Continue to roll your shoulders up off the floor, lifting your chin and extending your ears away from your shoulders (pictured).

○ Take a couple of breaths in the raised position before rolling slowly back to the floor.

○ Gradually increase the number of breaths at the top of the move, or repeat the sequence a couple of times.

Quick tip!
Don't push your hands into the floor to lift your head and shoulders, use your back muscles instead. Keep your shoulders relaxed and down.

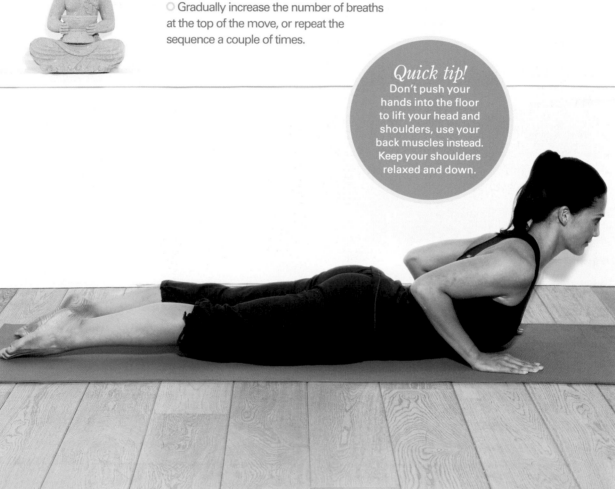

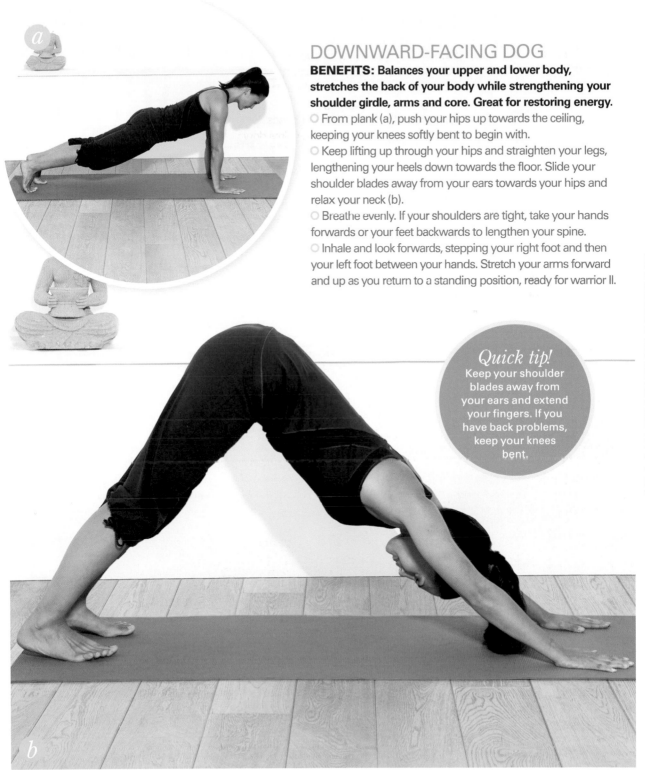

DOWNWARD-FACING DOG

BENEFITS: Balances your upper and lower body, stretches the back of your body while strengthening your shoulder girdle, arms and core. Great for restoring energy.

○ From plank (a), push your hips up towards the ceiling, keeping your knees softly bent to begin with.

○ Keep lifting up through your hips and straighten your legs, lengthening your heels down towards the floor. Slide your shoulder blades away from your ears towards your hips and relax your neck (b).

○ Breathe evenly. If your shoulders are tight, take your hands forwards or your feet backwards to lengthen your spine.

○ Inhale and look forwards, stepping your right foot and then your left foot between your hands. Stretch your arms forward and up as you return to a standing position, ready for warrior II.

Quick tip!
Keep your shoulder blades away from your ears and extend your fingers. If you have back problems, keep your knees bent.

MORNING ENERGISER MOVES

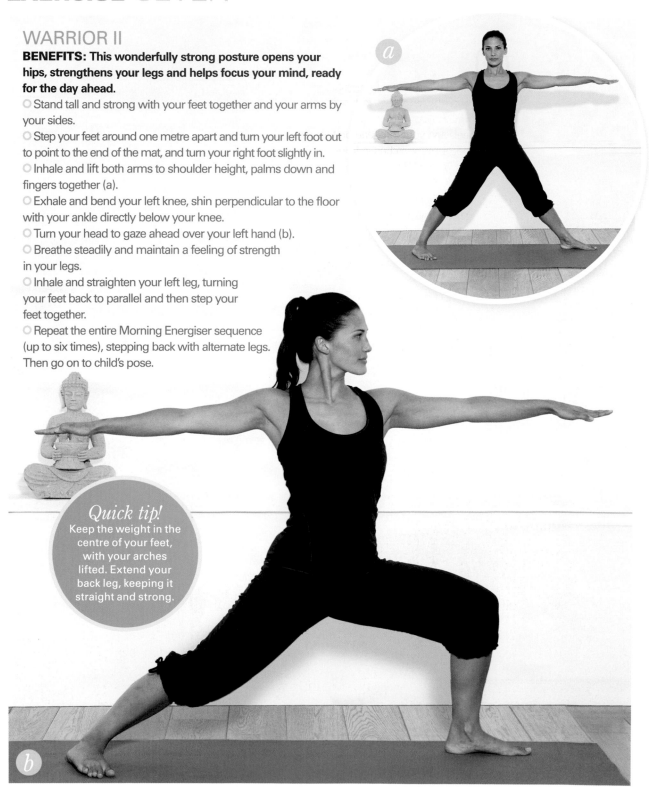

WARRIOR II

BENEFITS: This wonderfully strong posture opens your hips, strengthens your legs and helps focus your mind, ready for the day ahead.

○ Stand tall and strong with your feet together and your arms by your sides.

○ Step your feet around one metre apart and turn your left foot out to point to the end of the mat, and turn your right foot slightly in.

○ Inhale and lift both arms to shoulder height, palms down and fingers together (a).

○ Exhale and bend your left knee, shin perpendicular to the floor with your ankle directly below your knee.

○ Turn your head to gaze ahead over your left hand (b).

○ Breathe steadily and maintain a feeling of strength in your legs.

○ Inhale and straighten your left leg, turning your feet back to parallel and then step your feet together.

○ Repeat the entire Morning Energiser sequence (up to six times), stepping back with alternate legs. Then go on to child's pose.

Quick tip!
Keep the weight in the centre of your feet, with your arches lifted. Extend your back leg, keeping it straight and strong.

CHILD'S POSE

BENEFITS: A relaxing posture to gently lengthen your spine.

○ Place your bottom on your heels and your forehead on the floor, arms stretched in front of you, palms facing down. Rest for five to 10 breaths before turning over to lie on your back, legs shoulder-width apart, for a couple of minutes. Allow your body to absorb the feeling of stillness before heading off and having a wonderful day!

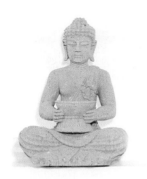

MORNING ENERGISER MOVES

Quick tip! Let your shoulders drop towards the floor. Imagine your back is expanding with your breath.

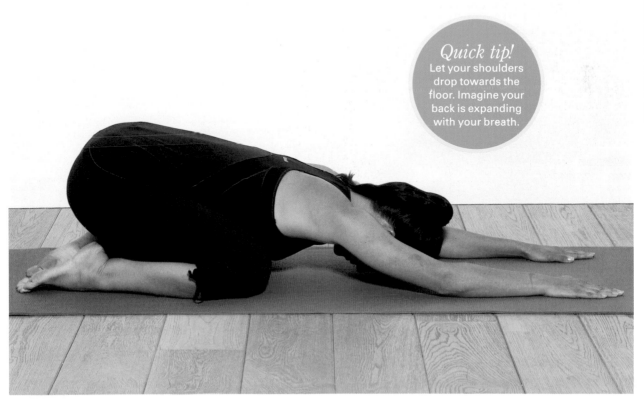

MORNING ENERGISER CIRCUIT

Sun salutations can be practised every day, but do them at least for two to three times a week. As you gain experience and become more familiar with the sequence, give more

1 STANDING
FORWARD BEND
PAGE 40

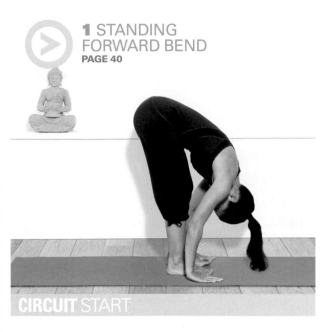

CIRCUIT START

2 LUNGE
WARRIOR
PAGE 41

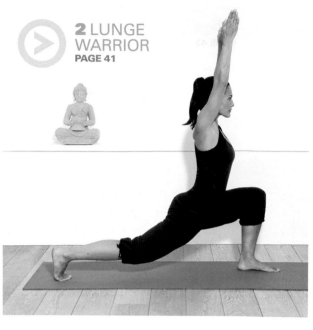

8 CHILD'S POSE
PAGE 47

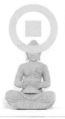

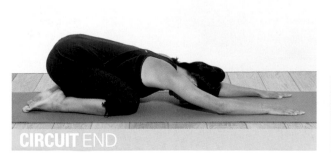

CIRCUIT END

7 WARRIOR II
PAGE 46

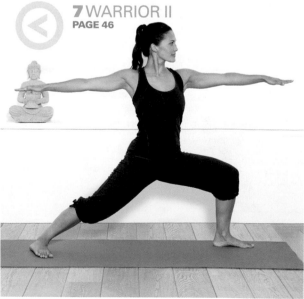

attention to your breath. Breathing through your nose warms and filters the air and helps slow your breathing down, bringing a meditative quality to your practice.

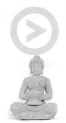

3 PLANK
PAGE 42

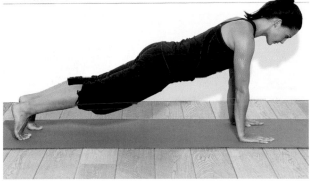

4 CROCODILE
PAGE 43

6 DOWNWARD-FACING DOG
PAGE 45

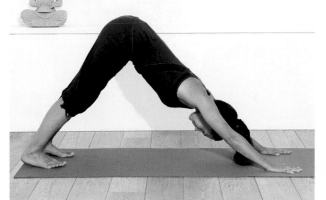

5 COBRA
PAGE 44

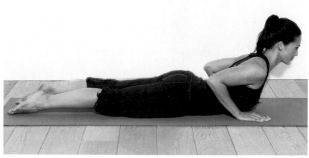

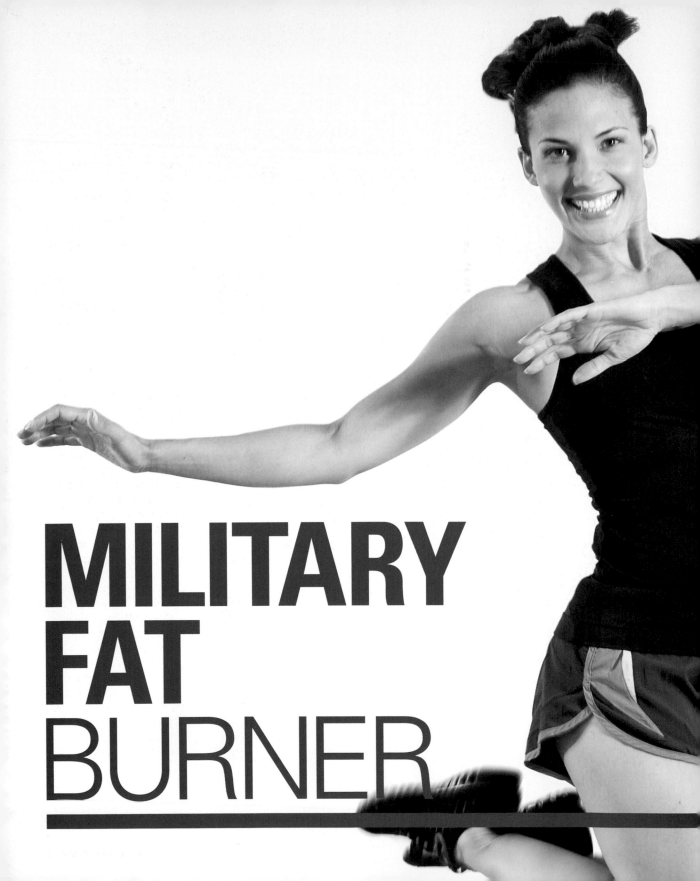

MILITARY
FAT
BURNER

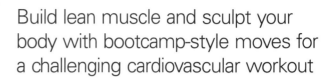

MILITARY FAT BURNER

Build lean muscle and sculpt your body with bootcamp-style moves for a challenging cardiovascular workout

Military-style **exercises are hugely popular at the moment and that's because they work! This routine is designed to challenge your cardiovascular system (see page 18) to burn calories and fat. When you use a medicine ball and a kettlebell it makes a significant demand on your muscles, helping you build lean muscle tissue and sculpt a defined physique. If you use a combination of anaerobic exercise (short, intense bursts of exercise that increase muscle strength) and weight training you boost your metabolism even further, which is a great way to help you get in shape.**

Anaerobic exercise usually involves intense bursts that use your whole body, plus power and speed. The increased effort pushes your heart rate up very high.

The exercises take the form of interval training, which challenges your anaerobic fitness system, burning fat and improving your fitness levels. The exercises used here also work against resistance, taking care of all of your fitness needs in one go!

You'll use a medicine ball and kettlebell for some of these exercises, but if you don't have them, you can still benefit. For the medicine ball exercises, simply hold a single dumbbell, one end in each hand. For the squat thrust, place your hands on the floor instead.

If you don't own a kettlebell, you can repeat the burpee move (that should encourage you to go out and buy one!).

This circuit will help strengthen your entire body, building muscle definition as well as torching calories. Make sure you stretch thoroughly afterwards to avoid muscle soreness.

MILITARY FAT BURNER MOVES

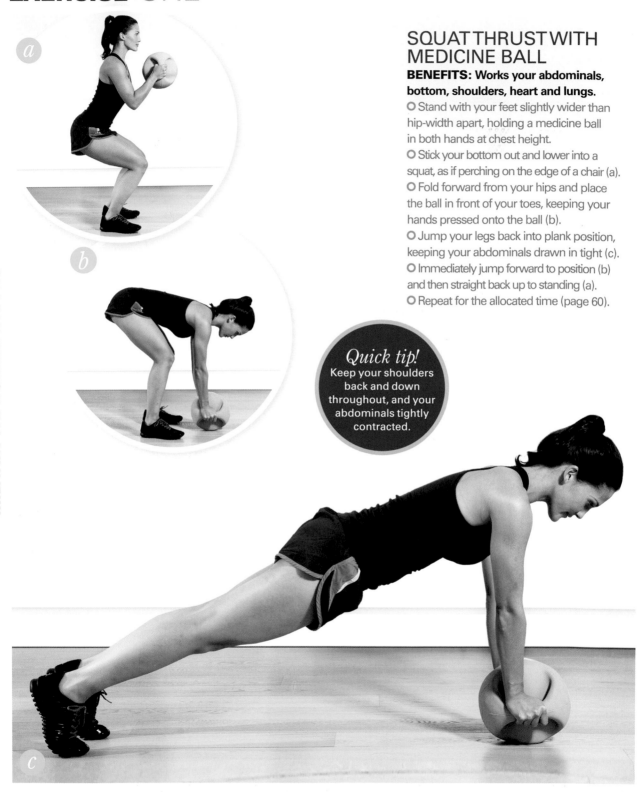

a

b

c

SQUAT THRUST WITH MEDICINE BALL

BENEFITS: Works your abdominals, bottom, shoulders, heart and lungs.

○ Stand with your feet slightly wider than hip-width apart, holding a medicine ball in both hands at chest height.

○ Stick your bottom out and lower into a squat, as if perching on the edge of a chair (a).

○ Fold forward from your hips and place the ball in front of your toes, keeping your hands pressed onto the ball (b).

○ Jump your legs back into plank position, keeping your abdominals drawn in tight (c).

○ Immediately jump forward to position (b) and then straight back up to standing (a).

○ Repeat for the allocated time (page 60).

Quick tip!
Keep your shoulders back and down throughout, and your abdominals tightly contracted.

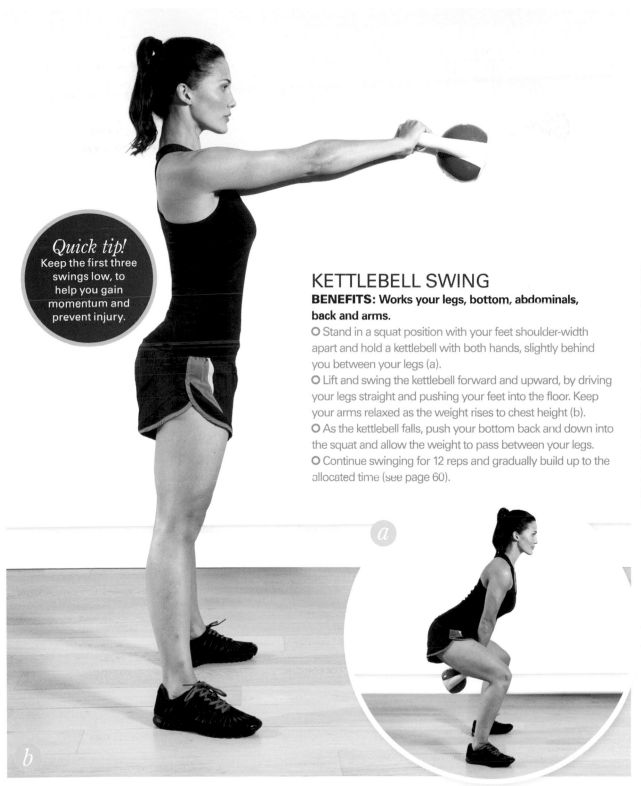

Quick tip!
Keep the first three swings low, to help you gain momentum and prevent injury.

KETTLEBELL SWING

BENEFITS: Works your legs, bottom, abdominals, back and arms.

O Stand in a squat position with your feet shoulder-width apart and hold a kettlebell with both hands, slightly behind you between your legs (a).

O Lift and swing the kettlebell forward and upward, by driving your legs straight and pushing your feet into the floor. Keep your arms relaxed as the weight rises to chest height (b).

O As the kettlebell falls, push your bottom back and down into the squat and allow the weight to pass between your legs.

O Continue swinging for 12 reps and gradually build up to the allocated time (see page 60).

a

b

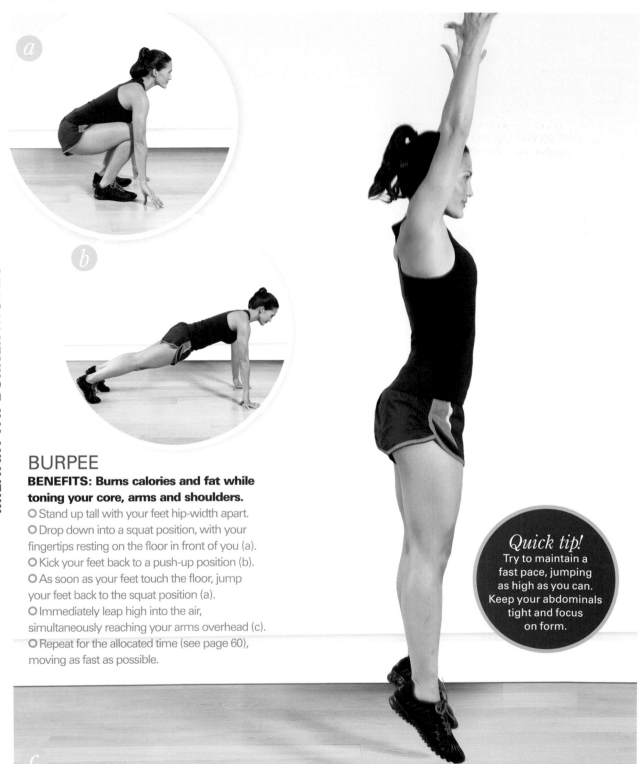

MILITARY FAT BURNER MOVES

BURPEE

BENEFITS: Burns calories and fat while toning your core, arms and shoulders.

- Stand up tall with your feet hip-width apart.
- Drop down into a squat position, with your fingertips resting on the floor in front of you (a).
- Kick your feet back to a push-up position (b).
- As soon as your feet touch the floor, jump your feet back to the squat position (a).
- Immediately leap high into the air, simultaneously reaching your arms overhead (c).
- Repeat for the allocated time (see page 60), moving as fast as possible.

Quick tip!
Try to maintain a fast pace, jumping as high as you can. Keep your abdominals tight and focus on form.

KNEE DRIVER WITH MEDICINE BALL

BENEFITS: Great for toning your abdominals, back and shoulders. Also challenges your cardiovascular system.

O Start in plank position with a straight, neutral spine, resting on your toes with your hands pressing onto the medicine ball (a).

O Bend your right knee and drive it in toward your chest (b).

O Jump your right leg back as you drive your left knee toward your chest.

O Alternate your legs in a running motion for the allocated time (see page 60) without resting, so only one foot is in contact with the floor at a time.

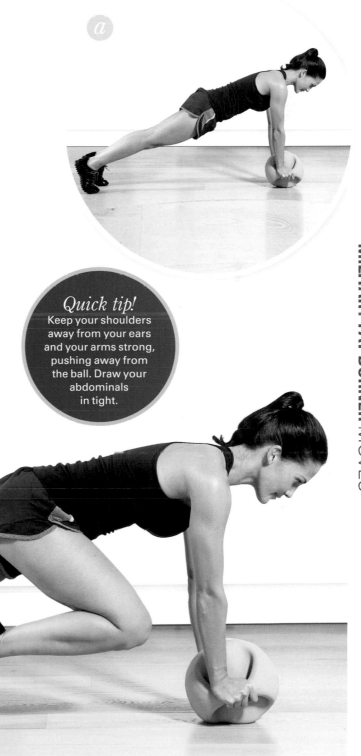

Quick tip!
Keep your shoulders away from your ears and your arms strong, pushing away from the ball. Draw your abdominals in tight.

MILITARY FAT BURNER MOVES

MILITARY FAT BURNER MOVES

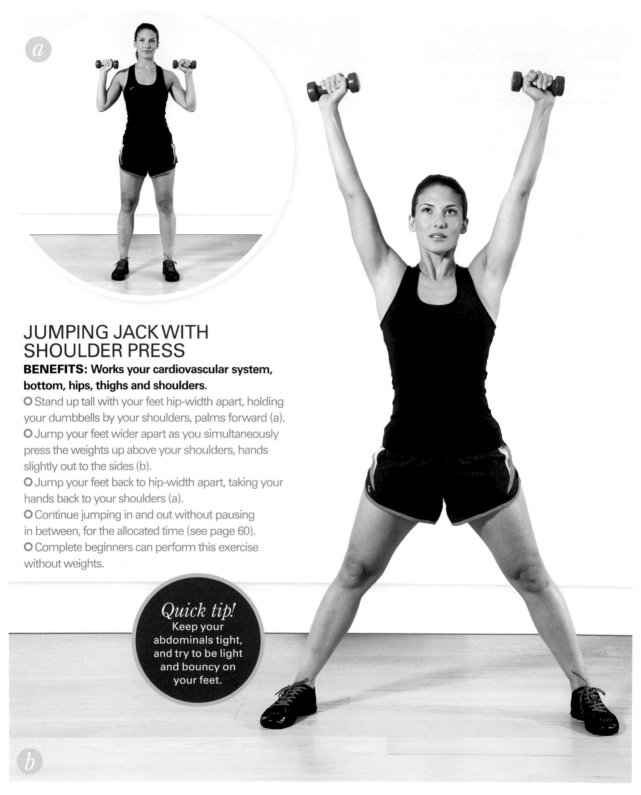

a

JUMPING JACK WITH SHOULDER PRESS

BENEFITS: Works your cardiovascular system, bottom, hips, thighs and shoulders.

O Stand up tall with your feet hip-width apart, holding your dumbbells by your shoulders, palms forward (a).

O Jump your feet wider apart as you simultaneously press the weights up above your shoulders, hands slightly out to the sides (b).

O Jump your feet back to hip-width apart, taking your hands back to your shoulders (a).

O Continue jumping in and out without pausing in between, for the allocated time (see page 60).

O Complete beginners can perform this exercise without weights.

Quick tip!
Keep your abdominals tight, and try to be light and bouncy on your feet.

b

PRESS-UP

BENEFITS: Strengthens your chest, upper arms and core.

○ Start on your hands and toes, with your body forming a straight line and your abdominals drawn in (a).

○ Bend your elbows and lower your body in a straight line towards the floor (b).

○ Exhale and push back up to position (a).

○ On your second circuit (see page 60), change your arm position so your hands are close together, fingers spread out, a diamond shape between your thumbs and index fingers. Repeat for the allocated time.

○ Beginners can perform press-ups on their knees with their ankles crossed. Lower the whole of your upper torso towards the floor, not just your head.

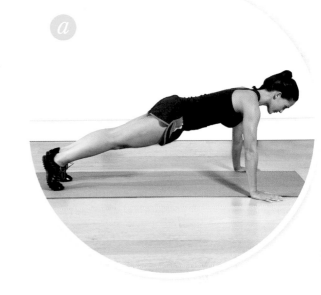

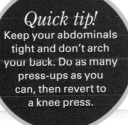

Quick tip!
Keep your abdominals tight and don't arch your back. Do as many press-ups as you can, then revert to a knee press.

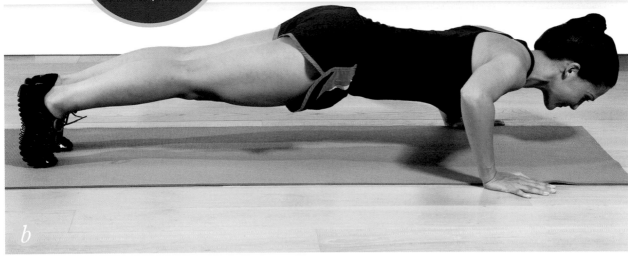

MILITARY FAT BURNER MOVES

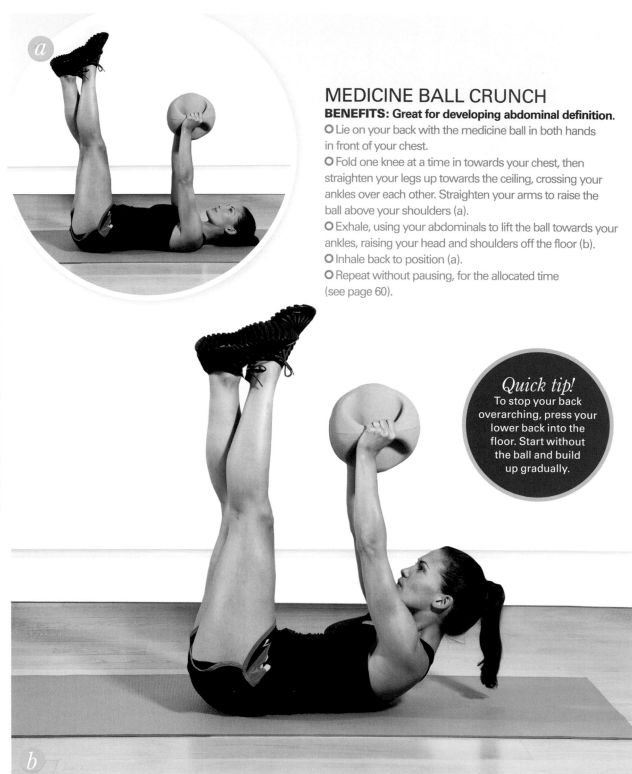

MILITARY FAT BURNER MOVES

MEDICINE BALL CRUNCH

BENEFITS: Great for developing abdominal definition.

O Lie on your back with the medicine ball in both hands in front of your chest.

O Fold one knee at a time in towards your chest, then straighten your legs up towards the ceiling, crossing your ankles over each other. Straighten your arms to raise the ball above your shoulders (a).

O Exhale, using your abdominals to lift the ball towards your ankles, raising your head and shoulders off the floor (b).

O Inhale back to position (a).

O Repeat without pausing, for the allocated time (see page 60).

Quick tip!
To stop your back overarching, press your lower back into the floor. Start without the ball and build up gradually.

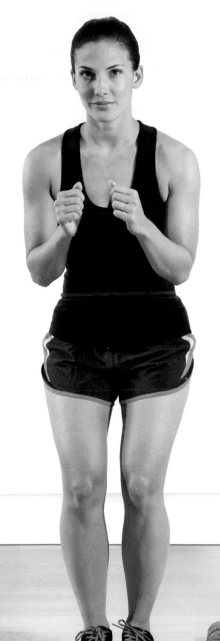

TOWEL JUMP

BENEFITS: Challenges your heart and lungs and strengthens your legs.

○ Roll up a towel and place it on the floor.
○ Stand to one side of the towel.
○ Jump back and forth across the towel for the allocated time (see page 60).

Quick tip!
Stay light on your feet. Try to be as quiet as possible and keep your abdominals tight.

MILITARY FAT BURNER MOVES

MILITARY FAT BURNER CIRCUIT

Beginners should start with a single circuit – 30 seconds per exercise with a one-minute recovery in between. As your fitness and stamina improve, build up to two circuits – one

1 SQUAT THRUST WITH MEDICINE BALL
PAGE 52

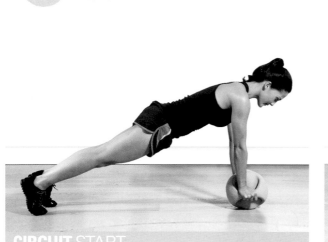

CIRCUIT START

2 KETTLEBELL SWING
PAGE 53

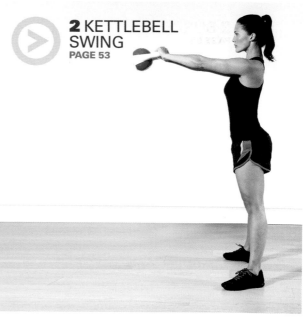

8 TOWEL JUMP
PAGE 59

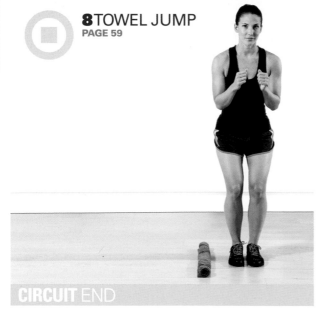

CIRCUIT END

7 MEDICINE BALL CRUNCH
PAGE 58

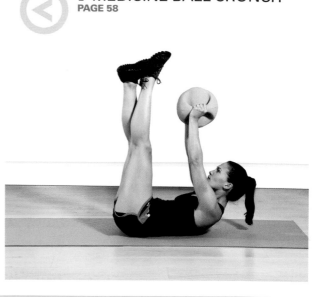

minute per exercise, with shorter rests between. Eventually, aim for three circuits of one minute per exercise. If you want to lose weight, do this workout three times a week. For general conditioning, mix it into your routine once a week, or use it as one of your cardiovascular sessions.

 3 BURPEE
PAGE 54

 4 KNEE DRIVER WITH MEDICINE BALL
PAGE 55

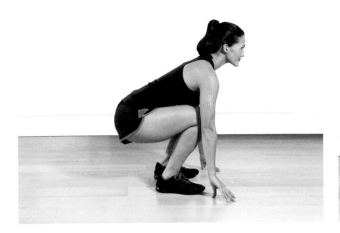

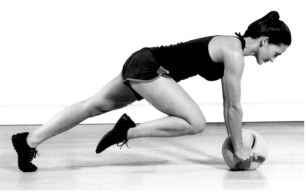

 6 PRESS-UP
PAGE 57

5 JUMPING JACK WITH SHOULDER PRESS
PAGE 56

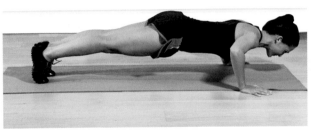

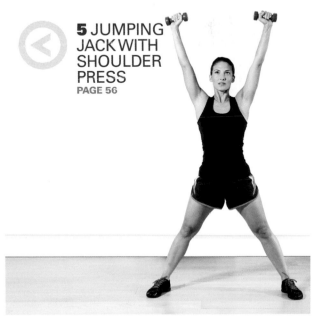

MILITARY FAT BURNER CIRCUIT

LOWER
BODY
BLAST

Beat cellulite and tone up your bum with a routine that slims your thighs and adds definition to your figure

Saddle bags, **wobbly thighs, pear-shaped body. We all have pet hates about our lower half. If you want to tone up your bum and thighs, these moves will do the trick.**

Unfortunately, women are pre-disposed to lay down fat on their lower body for fertility. The good news is, this fat is not as dangerous for your health as fat around your middle, and the even better news is there are plenty of great exercises to help reduce it.

The following exercises, combined with your cardiovascular workouts, will help lift your bottom, slim your hips and tone and define your thighs.

If you're a pear shape, working on adding definition to your shoulders can help balance out your proportions. If cellulite is your lower-body pet hate, remember this annoying orange peel is just a visible form of fat, so exercising will make all the difference. You can also tackle cellulite from the inside, by drinking plenty of water and avoiding coffee, alcohol and other common toxins, such as trans fats and additives.

Although you're probably already conscious of your food and fat intake, it's important to eat enough good quality fat, as this will help improve the quality of your cells. Good fats include avocado, olive oil and fish oils, and can be taken in supplement form or as part of a healthy diet.

Another top tip for toned legs is to body brush daily: by brushing your skin with firm strokes in an upwards direction, you can stimulate your circulation and help cleanse your body.

This routine is fantastic for anybody who wants lean, strong and defined legs and bum. All you need is an exercise band!

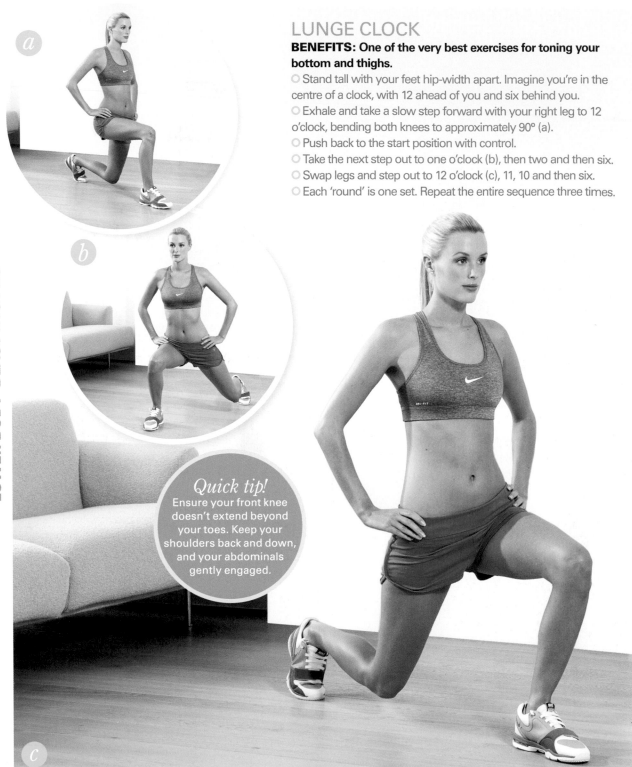

LUNGE CLOCK

BENEFITS: One of the very best exercises for toning your bottom and thighs.

○ Stand tall with your feet hip-width apart. Imagine you're in the centre of a clock, with 12 ahead of you and six behind you.

○ Exhale and take a slow step forward with your right leg to 12 o'clock, bending both knees to approximately 90º (a).

○ Push back to the start position with control.

○ Take the next step out to one o'clock (b), then two and then six.

○ Swap legs and step out to 12 o'clock (c), 11, 10 and then six.

○ Each 'round' is one set. Repeat the entire sequence three times.

Quick tip!

Ensure your front knee doesn't extend beyond your toes. Keep your shoulders back and down, and your abdominals gently engaged.

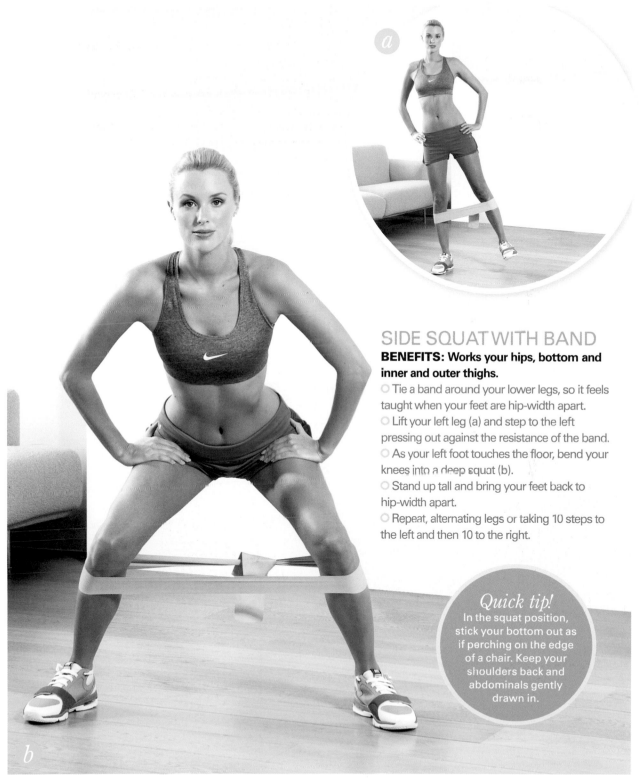

SIDE SQUAT WITH BAND

BENEFITS: Works your hips, bottom and inner and outer thighs.

○ Tie a band around your lower legs, so it feels taught when your feet are hip-width apart.

○ Lift your left leg (a) and step to the left pressing out against the resistance of the band.

○ As your left foot touches the floor, bend your knees into a deep squat (b).

○ Stand up tall and bring your feet back to hip-width apart.

○ Repeat, alternating legs or taking 10 steps to the left and then 10 to the right.

Quick tip!

In the squat position, stick your bottom out as if perching on the edge of a chair. Keep your shoulders back and abdominals gently drawn in.

SIDE PRESS

BENEFITS: Works your outer hip and thigh on your moving leg and your gluteals on both legs.

○ Tie the band around your legs just below your knees, so it feels slightly tight when your feet are shoulder-width apart.

○ Lift your right foot off the ground and press out against the band 10 times.

○ Try to balance on your supporting leg or, if necessary, lean against a wall or chair.

○ Repeat with your left leg.

LOWER BODY BLAST MOVES

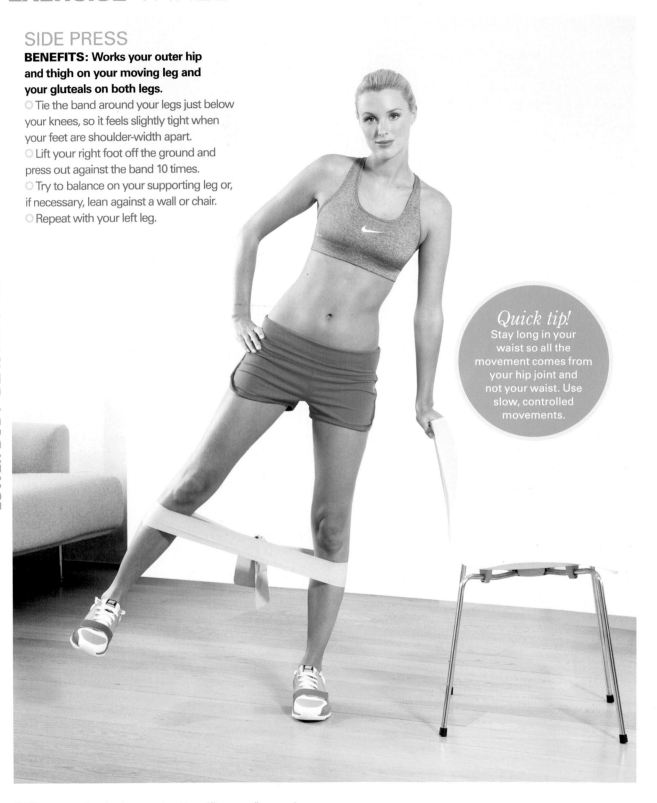

Quick tip!
Stay long in your waist so all the movement comes from your hip joint and not your waist. Use slow, controlled movements.

HIP LIFT WITH BAND

BENEFITS: Works your bottom and the back of your thighs.

○ Lie on your back with your knees bent and the band tied around your knees (a).

○ Squeeze your bottom to lift your hips up into the air (b).

○ Keeping your hips raised, push your knees out against the band four times.

○ Lower your hips back to the floor, then repeat six times.

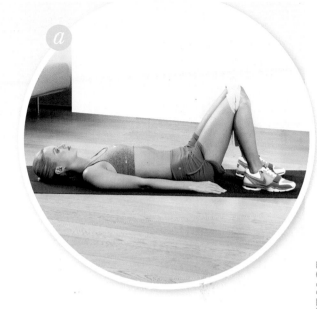

Quick tip!
Tuck your tailbone under as you lift your hips to help engage your bottom muscles.

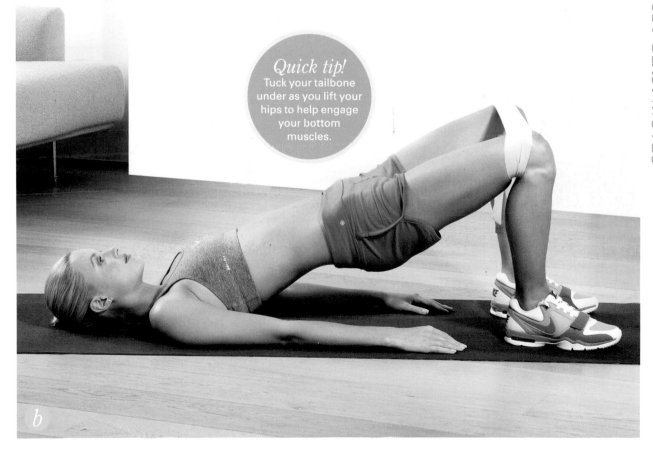

LOWER BODY BLAST MOVES

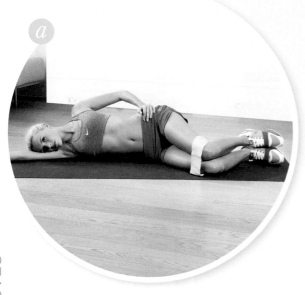

a

CLAM SHELL

BENEFITS: Works your bottom and deep hip rotator muscles.

○ Lie on your right side, with your head on your outstretched right arm, left hand on your hip. Bend both legs, with the band tied around your knees (a).

○ Exhale and raise your left knee like a clam against the resistance of the band, keeping your feet together (b).

○ Inhale to close.

○ Repeat 15 times on each side. On the last rep, hold in the open position and pulse 15 times.

LOWER BODY **BLAST** MOVES

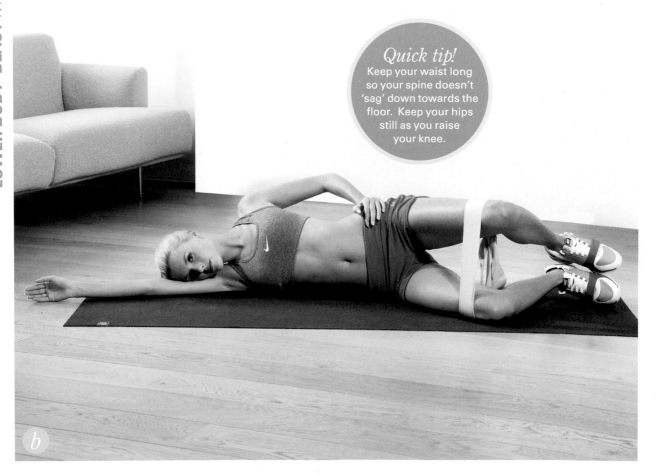

b

Quick tip!
Keep your waist long so your spine doesn't 'sag' down towards the floor. Keep your hips still as you raise your knee.

SINGLE LEG PRESS

BENEFITS: Works your bottom, legs and core stabilising muscles.

○ Lie on your back, with your left knee bent, foot flat on the floor and your right knee above your hip, foot in the band, pulling the ends of the band tight, one end in each hand (a).

○ Inhale to prepare, exhale and engage your abdominals as you push your right leg forward and up into the band (b).

○ Inhale and slowly return to position (a).

○ Repeat 10 times on each leg.

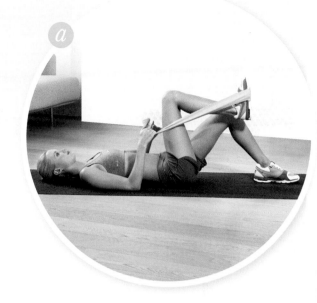

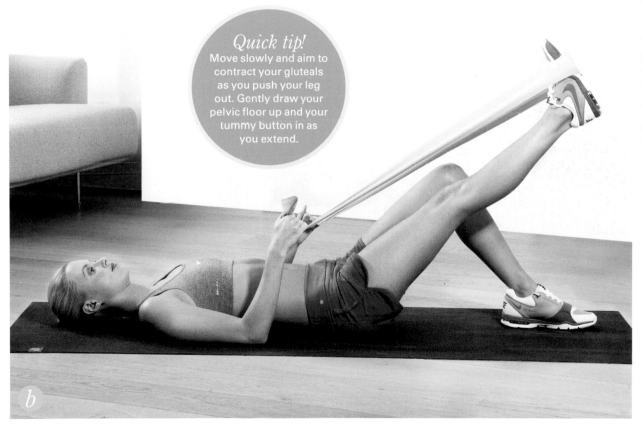

Quick tip!
Move slowly and aim to contract your gluteals as you push your leg out. Gently draw your pelvic floor up and your tummy button in as you extend.

LOWER BODY BLAST MOVES

DONKEY KICK

BENEFITS: A great exercise for lifting your bottom and giving definition.

○ Start on all fours then lower yourself onto your forearms, hands clasped together.

○ Extend your right leg behind you, while keeping your hips level and your spine in neutral (a).

○ Exhale to lift your leg higher (b), inhale to lower.

○ Perform 12 reps, followed by 12 pulses at the top position.

○ Repeat the above exercise with a bent knee (c).

○ Perform 12 reps.

○ Repeat the entire series on the left leg.

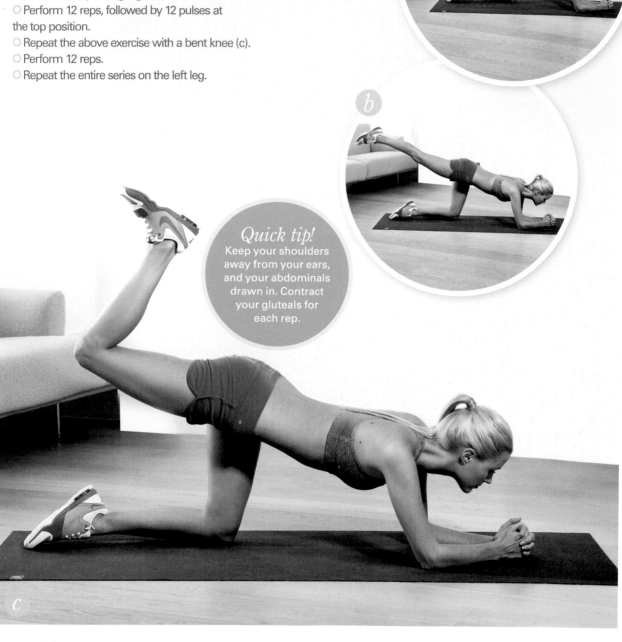

Quick tip!
Keep your shoulders away from your ears, and your abdominals drawn in. Contract your gluteals for each rep.

SIDE LEG LIFT

BENEFITS: These Pilates leg exercises work on the small muscles to help strengthen and define your bottom and thighs.

○ Lie on your right side with your head on your outstretched right arm, your left leg on top of your right leg, left hand on your left hip.

○ Keep your spine straight and your lower waist lifted, as you lengthen your left leg (a).

○ Exhale as you lift your left leg, keeping your hips and waist still (b), and inhale to lower.

○ Perform 15 reps, then repeat on the other side.

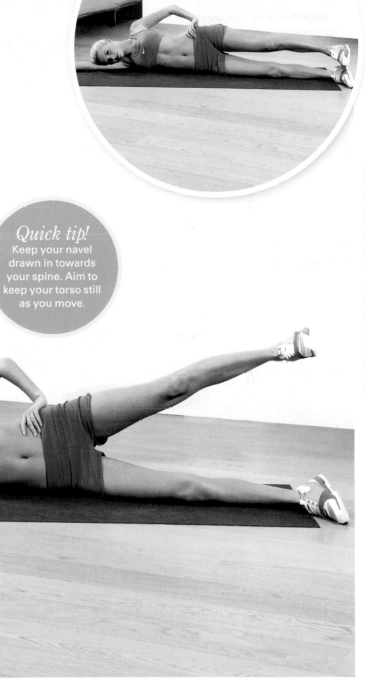

a

Quick tip!
Keep your navel drawn in towards your spine. Aim to keep your torso still as you move.

b

LOWER BODY BLAST MOVES

LOWER BODY BLAST CIRCUIT

If your lower body is your problem area, try to perform these exercises twice a week, as well as your cardiovascular work and one other resistance session of your choice.

1 LUNGE CLOCK
REPS: 3 ON EACH LEG
PAGE 64

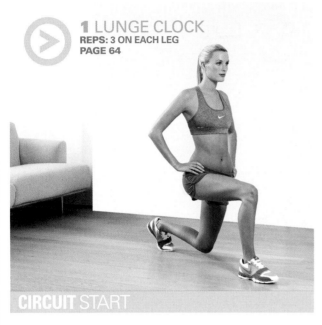

CIRCUIT START

2 SIDE SQUAT WITH BAND
REPS: 10 TO EACH SIDE
PAGE 65

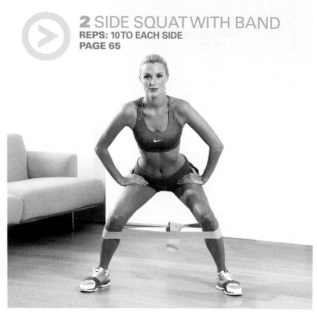

8 SIDE LEG LIFT
REPS: 15 ON EACH LEG
PAGE 71

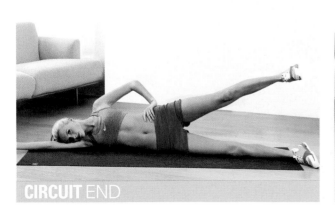

CIRCUIT END

7 DONKEY KICK
REPS: 12 ON EACH LEG
PAGE 70

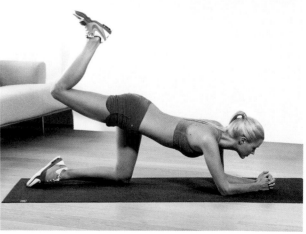

3 SIDE PRESS
REPS: 10 ON EACH LEG
PAGE 66

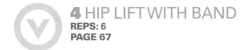

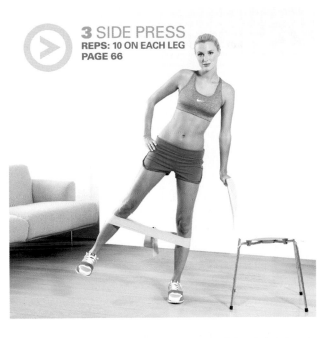

4 HIP LIFT WITH BAND
REPS: 6
PAGE 67

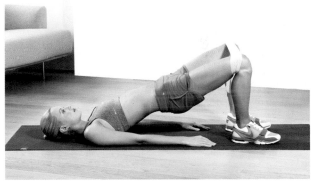

6 SINGLE LEG PRESS
REPS: 10 ON EACH LEG
PAGE 09

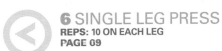

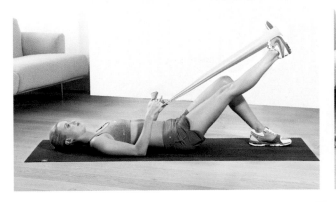

5 CLAM SHELL
REPS: 15 ON EACH LEG
PAGE 68

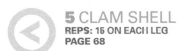

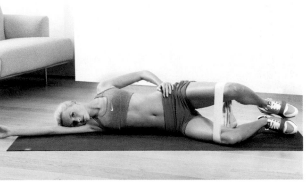

LOWER BODY BLAST CIRCUIT

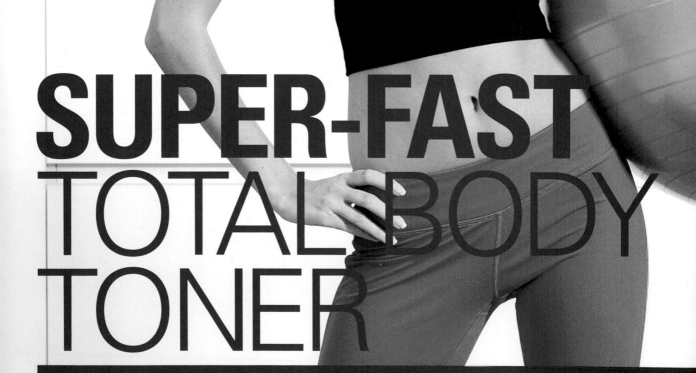

SUPER-FAST
TOTAL BODY
TONER

SUPER-FAST
TOTAL BODY TONER

Work your whole body in just eight super-powerful moves

In our fast-paced lives every second counts, so this routine has been designed to give you a total body workout in just 12 minutes.

The exercises here are known as 'compound moves' which means they work more than one joint or muscle group at the same time. This means your heart has to work a little harder to supply blood to your working muscles, while you can reduce the length of your workout by training two areas simultaneously.

These moves are all resistance exercises, simply meaning that your muscles have to work against a resistance to create a movement. You'll need a set of dumbbells to perform them, but if you don't want to commit to purchasing dumbbells just yet, you could always fill a couple of 1–1.5-litre bottles with sand or water for a similar effect. As we're targeting several muscle groups at the same time, you'll feel your heart rate increase, so your cardiovascular system will benefit too.

Remember, by increasing your muscle mass you'll boost your metabolism (the rate at which your body burns calories), because muscle tissue burns more calories than other body tissue, such as fat.

You don't have to be afraid of using weights, either. Women often worry about getting 'too big' or too masculine from weight training, but you have significantly less of the hormones required to build muscle mass than men do, so it's actually very difficult for you to get large and bulky through weight-training alone.

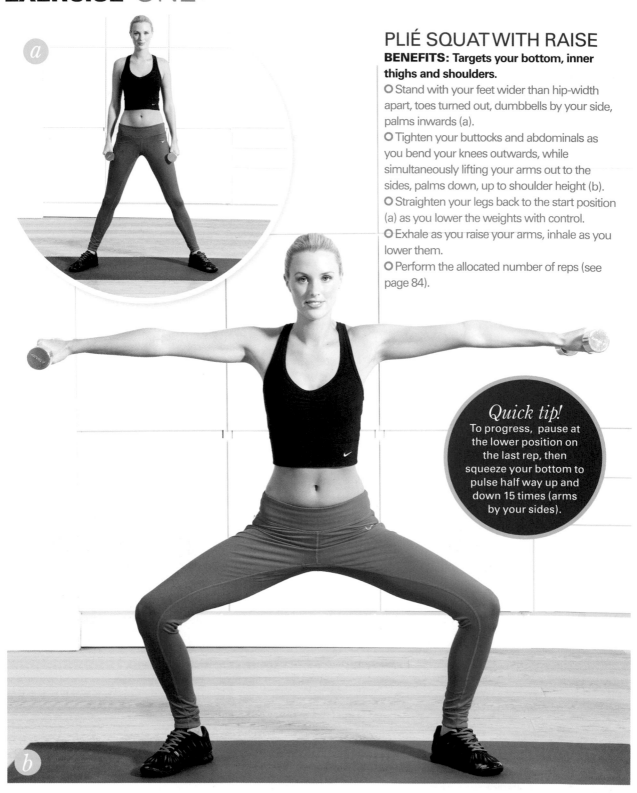

SUPER-FAST WORKOUT MOVES

PLIÉ SQUAT WITH RAISE

BENEFITS: **Targets your bottom, inner thighs and shoulders.**

O Stand with your feet wider than hip-width apart, toes turned out, dumbbells by your side, palms inwards (a).

O Tighten your buttocks and abdominals as you bend your knees outwards, while simultaneously lifting your arms out to the sides, palms down, up to shoulder height (b).

O Straighten your legs back to the start position (a) as you lower the weights with control.

O Exhale as you raise your arms, inhale as you lower them.

O Perform the allocated number of reps (see page 84).

Quick tip!
To progress, pause at the lower position on the last rep, then squeeze your bottom to pulse half way up and down 15 times (arms by your sides).

LUNGE TWIST WITH MEDICINE BALL

BENEFITS: Targets your bottom and thighs, plus your waist and shoulders.

O Stand tall with your feet close but not touching, the medicine ball held in front of your hips (a).

O Take a large step forward with your left leg and simultaneously bend both knees to an approximate right angle, as you raise the ball in front of you to shoulder height (b).

O In the lunge position, twist your torso and the ball to the left (c).

O Return to face forward, then step back to the start position.

O Alternate to the left and right for the allocated number of reps (see page 84).

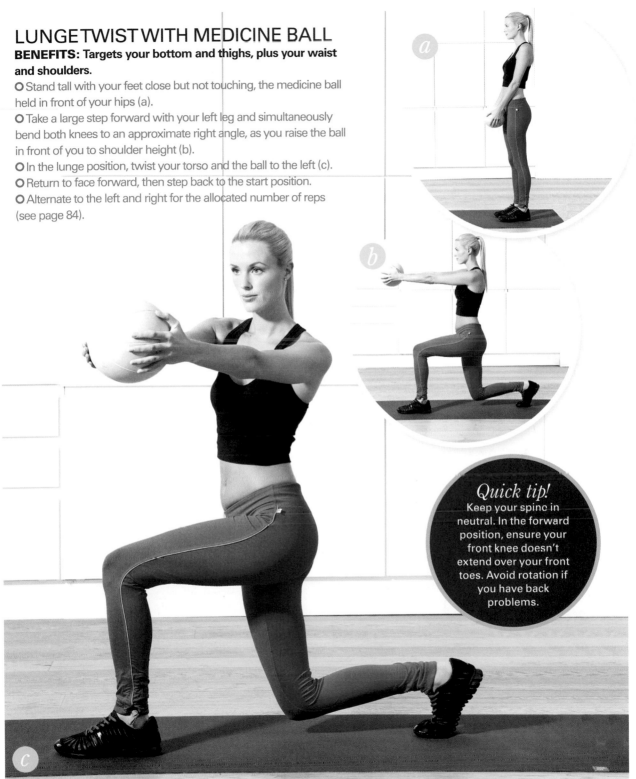

Quick tip!
Keep your spine in neutral. In the forward position, ensure your front knee doesn't extend over your front toes. Avoid rotation if you have back problems.

SUPER-FAST WORKOUT MOVES

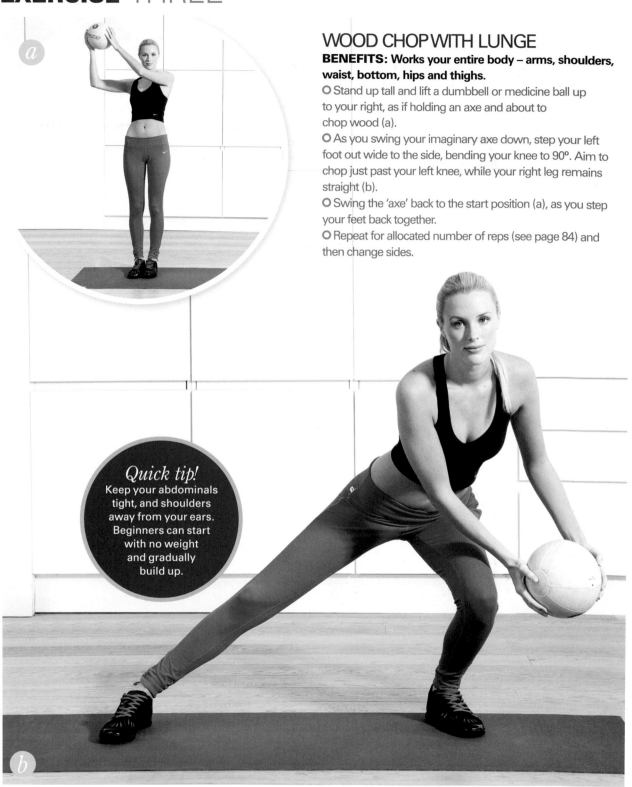

WOOD CHOP WITH LUNGE

BENEFITS: Works your entire body – arms, shoulders, waist, bottom, hips and thighs.

○ Stand up tall and lift a dumbbell or medicine ball up to your right, as if holding an axe and about to chop wood (a).

○ As you swing your imaginary axe down, step your left foot out wide to the side, bending your knee to 90º. Aim to chop just past your left knee, while your right leg remains straight (b).

○ Swing the 'axe' back to the start position (a), as you step your feet back together.

○ Repeat for allocated number of reps (see page 84) and then change sides.

Quick tip!
Keep your abdominals tight, and shoulders away from your ears. Beginners can start with no weight and gradually build up.

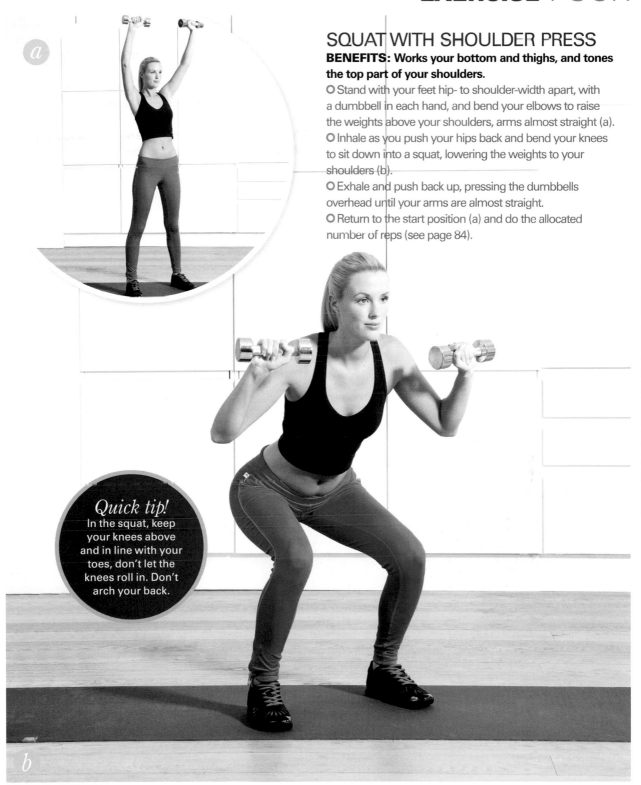

SQUAT WITH SHOULDER PRESS

BENEFITS: Works your bottom and thighs, and tones the top part of your shoulders.

O Stand with your feet hip- to shoulder-width apart, with a dumbbell in each hand, and bend your elbows to raise the weights above your shoulders, arms almost straight (a).

O Inhale as you push your hips back and bend your knees to sit down into a squat, lowering the weights to your shoulders (b).

O Exhale and push back up, pressing the dumbbells overhead until your arms are almost straight.

O Return to the start position (a) and do the allocated number of reps (see page 84).

Quick tip!
In the squat, keep your knees above and in line with your toes, don't let the knees roll in. Don't arch your back.

SUPER-FAST WORKOUT MOVES

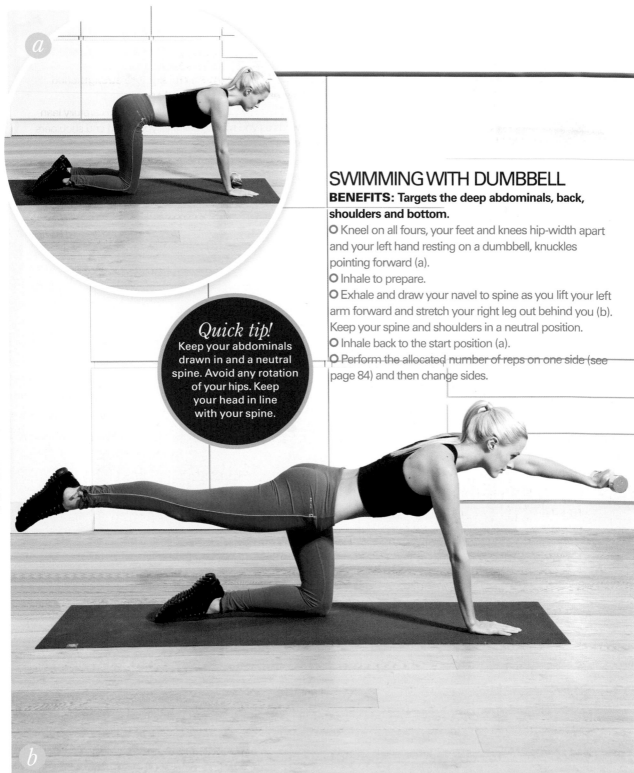

SUPER-FAST WORKOUT MOVES

a

SWIMMING WITH DUMBBELL

BENEFITS: Targets the deep abdominals, back, shoulders and bottom.

○ Kneel on all fours, your feet and knees hip-width apart and your left hand resting on a dumbbell, knuckles pointing forward (a).

○ Inhale to prepare.

○ Exhale and draw your navel to spine as you lift your left arm forward and stretch your right leg out behind you (b). Keep your spine and shoulders in a neutral position.

○ Inhale back to the start position (a).

○ Perform the allocated number of reps on one side (see page 84) and then change sides.

Quick tip!
Keep your abdominals drawn in and a neutral spine. Avoid any rotation of your hips. Keep your head in line with your spine.

b

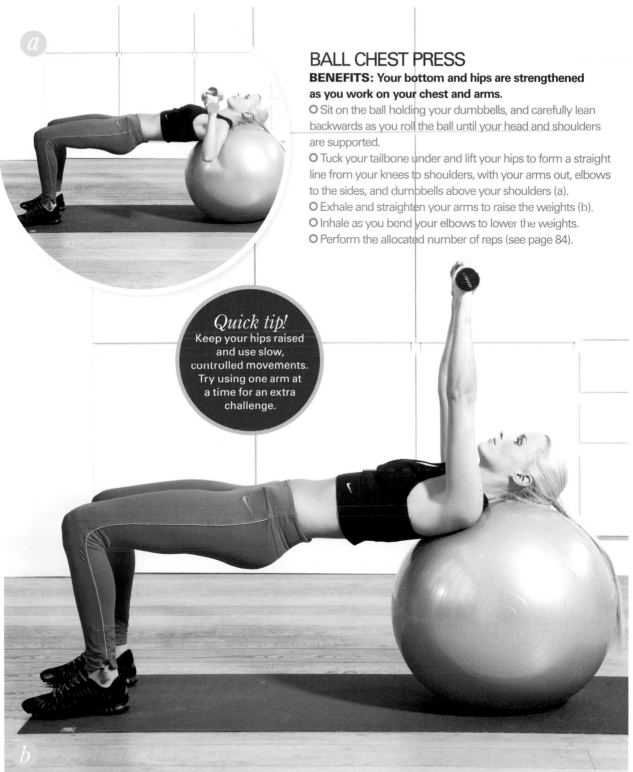

BALL CHEST PRESS

BENEFITS: Your bottom and hips are strengthened as you work on your chest and arms.

○ Sit on the ball holding your dumbbells, and carefully lean backwards as you roll the ball until your head and shoulders are supported.

○ Tuck your tailbone under and lift your hips to form a straight line from your knees to shoulders, with your arms out, elbows to the sides, and dumbbells above your shoulders (a).

○ Exhale and straighten your arms to raise the weights (b).

○ Inhale as you bend your elbows to lower the weights.

○ Perform the allocated number of reps (see page 84).

Quick tip!
Keep your hips raised and use slow, controlled movements. Try using one arm at a time for an extra challenge.

SUPER-FAST WORKOUT MOVES

SUPER-FAST WORKOUT MOVES

HIP LIFT

BENEFITS: Lifts and defines your bottom and back of your thighs

○ Lie on your back with your feet on top of an exercise ball, hands by your sides, palms facing down (a).

○ Exhale and squeeze your bottom, lifting your hips up in the air (b).

○ Inhale to lower half-way back down and continue smoothly onto the next hip lift.

○ As you advance, try a single-leg hip lift. Use the same technique, but extend and straighten one leg, keeping your thighs parallel. See page 84 for reps.

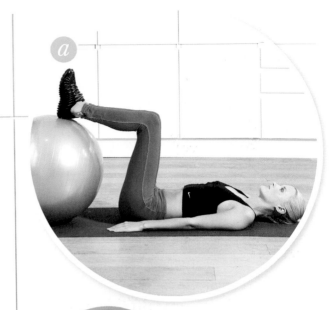

a

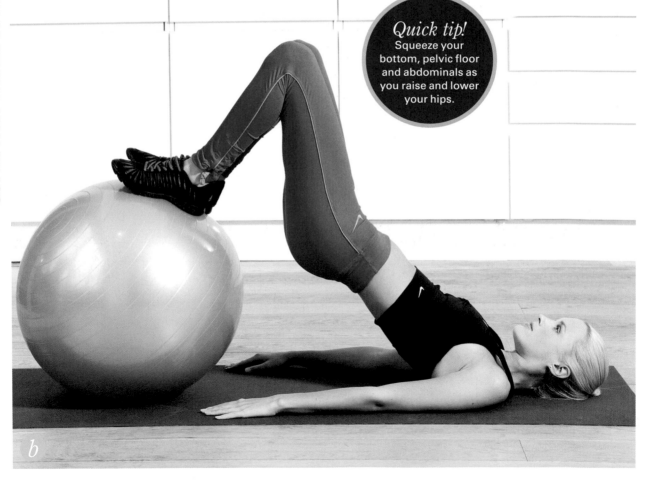

b

Quick tip!
Squeeze your bottom, pelvic floor and abdominals as you raise and lower your hips.

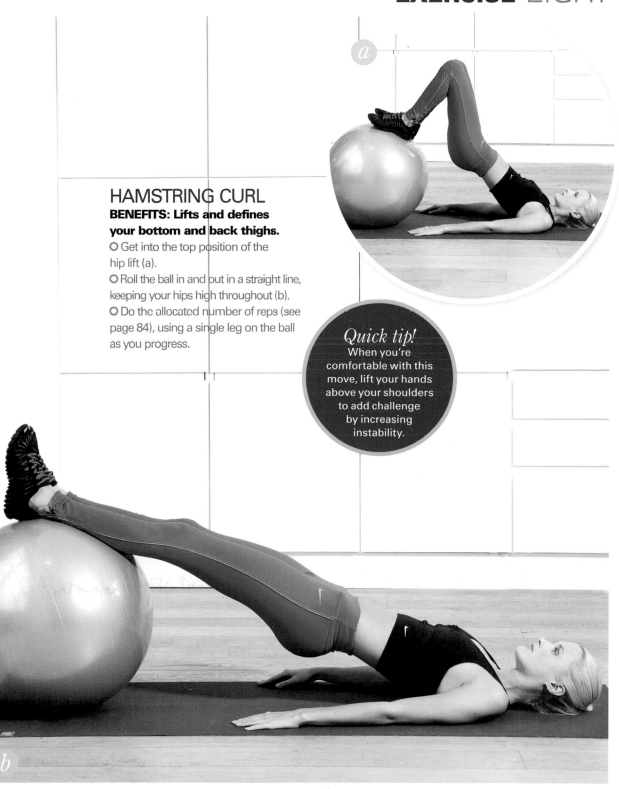

HAMSTRING CURL

**BENEFITS: Lifts and defines
your bottom and back thighs.**

O Get into the top position of the
hip lift (a).

O Roll the ball in and out in a straight line,
keeping your hips high throughout (b).

O Do the allocated number of reps (see
page 84), using a single leg on the ball
as you progress.

Quick tip!
When you're
comfortable with this
move, lift your hands
above your shoulders
to add challenge
by increasing
instability.

SUPER-FAST WORKOUT MOVES

SUPER-FAST TOTAL BODY TONER CIRCUIT

This workout is perfect to add into your routine when time is

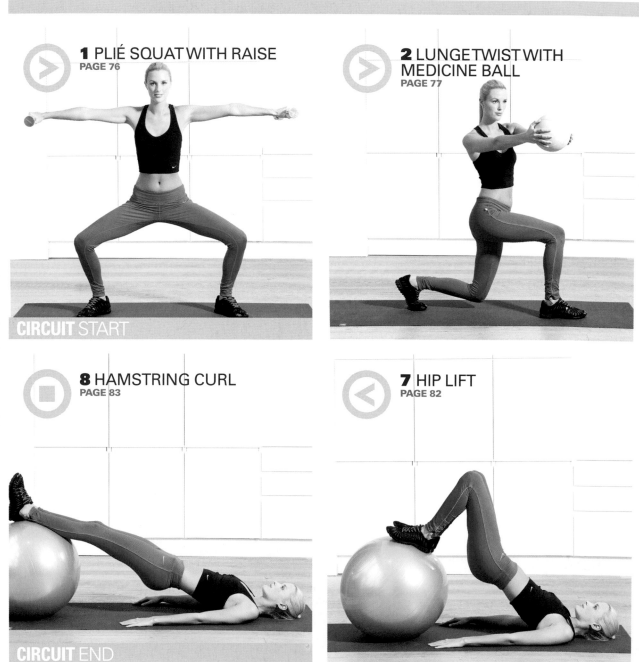

1 PLIÉ SQUAT WITH RAISE
PAGE 76

CIRCUIT START

2 LUNGE TWIST WITH MEDICINE BALL
PAGE 77

8 HAMSTRING CURL
PAGE 83

CIRCUIT END

7 HIP LIFT
PAGE 82

short. Alternatively, perform it at least twice a week as a stand-alone conditioning routine. Beginners should do 12–15 reps of each exercise, and build up to 15–20 reps.

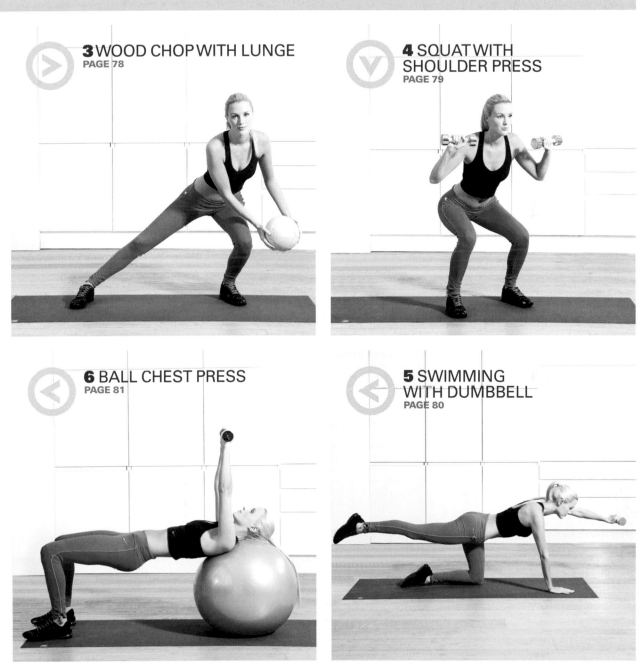

3 WOOD CHOP WITH LUNGE
PAGE 78

4 SQUAT WITH SHOULDER PRESS
PAGE 79

6 BALL CHEST PRESS
PAGE 81

5 SWIMMING WITH DUMBBELL
PAGE 80

SUPER-FAST WORKOUT CIRCUIT

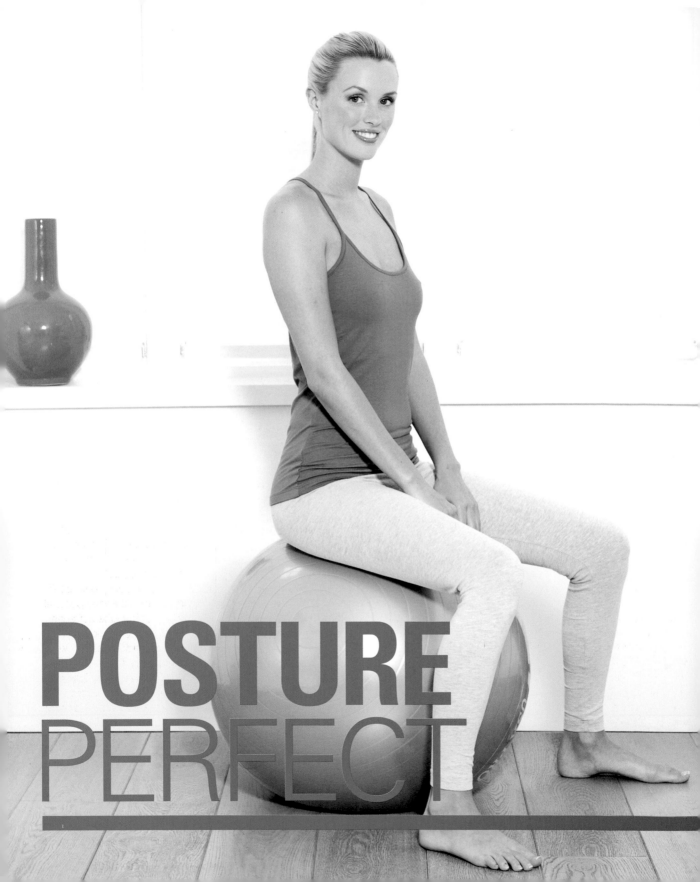

POSTURE
PERFECT

Look instantly slimmer and beat back pain with these postural moves

Life today isn't kind to your posture: working on computers and laptops tends to lead to a curved upper spine and rounded shoulders, as well as a 'head forward' position which can be uncomfortable and result in restricted mobility. Driving your car or sitting for long periods at a desk or in front of the TV also wreaks havoc on your spine, hamstrings and shoulders and can end up ruining your posture.

There are four types of postural alignment:
1) Ideal alignment – an 's'-shaped spine with a natural curve in the lower back.
2) Lordosis/kyphosis – an increased curve in the lower or upper back, with muscle tightness as a result.
3) Flat back – spinal curves are flattened and the pelvis is tipped backwards.
4) Sway back – the pelvis is tipped back, the upper spine is curved and the legs are slightly bent towards the back of the body.

This programme uses yoga and Pilates exercises to strengthen the muscles of the upper back and shoulder girdle, while stretching the chest muscles to help balance out excessively rounded shoulders and kyphosis.

We'll also focus on working the abdominals and deep core muscles of the torso to encourage a healthy neutral spine and reduce lordosis, as well as general stretches and conditioning to improve posture.

If you recognise yourself in any of the above postural types or if you're suffering from round shoulders, a 'hunch-back' posture or general tightness, practise the following exercises daily. Or you can select your favourite few and add them to any other workout, or include them at the end of your cardiovascular session.

POSTURE
TIPS

Stand sideways on to a mirror in your usual posture, then apply these clever tips and watch yourself grow taller and slimmer!

HEAD AND NECK
Try to create as much length as you can between your ears and shoulders. Imagine lengthening the crown (top) of your head towards the sky at all times.

TRANSVERSUS ABDOMINIS
Your core muscles are your own built-in corset. Just gently draw your navel to your spine to look pounds lighter!

SHOULDER GIRDLE
The shoulder girdle includes the top of your arms and your shoulder blades. For good shoulder posture, imagine you're sliding your shoulder blades down towards the back of your waist, opening your chest but without forcing the shoulders back in a 'sergeant major' fashion.

NEUTRAL SPINE
Your lower back should be neither arched, nor flattened, but somewhere in between.

LOWER BODY
With your weight in the centre of your feet, try to draw yourself up from your feet, as if creating space between the joints of your ankles, knees, pelvis and spine.

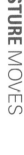

COBRA

BENEFITS: Strengthens your spine and helps counter round shoulders.

○ Lie face down, legs together, forehead on the floor and hands directly beneath your shoulders, palms down (a).

○ Inhale and slowly raise your forehead from the floor, followed by your nose and chin.

○ Continue to roll your shoulders off the floor, lifting your chin and keeping your shoulders away from your ears (b).

○ Take a couple of breaths at the top of the move before rolling slowly back to the floor.

○ Gradually increase the number of breaths or repeat the sequence a couple of times.

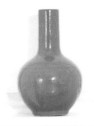

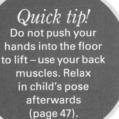

Quick tip!
Do not push your hands into the floor to lift – use your back muscles. Relax in child's pose afterwards (page 47).

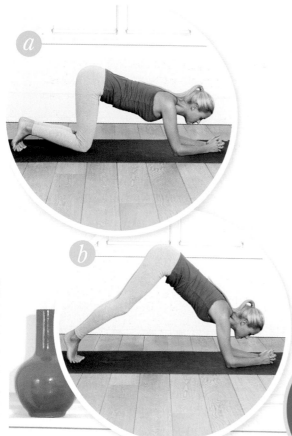

a

b

DOLPHIN

BENEFITS: Targets the muscles of your upper back, shoulders and shoulder blade stabilisers.

○ Lower down onto your knees and forearms, toes curled under. Clasp your hands together in front of you (a). To find the correct distance between your elbows, wrap the fingers of one hand around the opposite elbow.

○ Raise your hips towards the ceiling, so your body forms an inverted 'V' shape (b).

○ Inhale and rock your body forward so your chin comes over and in front of your hands (c).

○ Exhale to push back to the starting position (b) and repeat eight to 12 times.

Quick tip!
Keep your abdominals drawn in and your shoulder blades down. Beginners can start on their knees.

PERFECT POSTURE MOVES

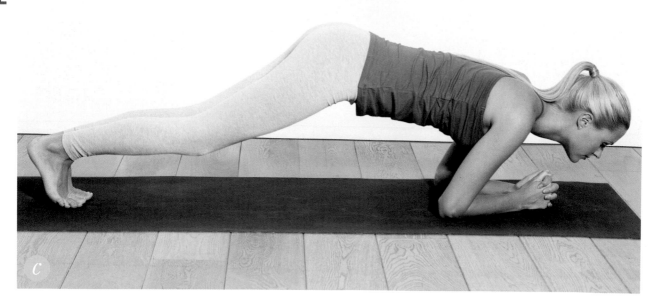

c

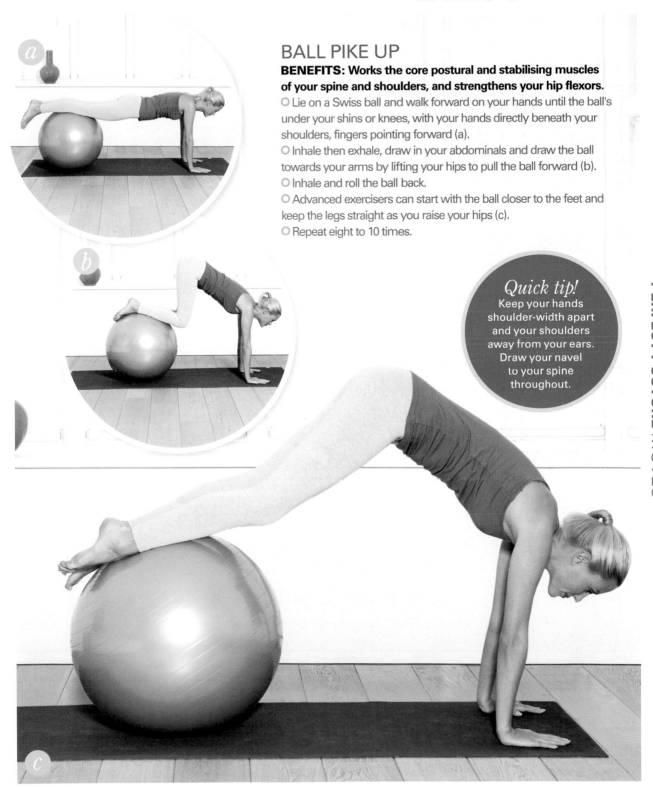

BALL PIKE UP

BENEFITS: Works the core postural and stabilising muscles of your spine and shoulders, and strengthens your hip flexors.

○ Lie on a Swiss ball and walk forward on your hands until the ball's under your shins or knees, with your hands directly beneath your shoulders, fingers pointing forward (a).

○ Inhale then exhale, draw in your abdominals and draw the ball towards your arms by lifting your hips to pull the ball forward (b).

○ Inhale and roll the ball back.

○ Advanced exercisers can start with the ball closer to the feet and keep the legs straight as you raise your hips (c).

○ Repeat eight to 10 times.

Quick tip!
Keep your hands shoulder-width apart and your shoulders away from your ears. Draw your navel to your spine throughout.

PERFECT POSTURE MOVES

PERFECT POSTURE MOVES

BALANCING STICK WITH TRICEPS PRESS

BENEFITS: Great for balance and postural muscles, specifically targeting your upper back, triceps, gluteals and core.

○ Stand with your feet hip-width apart, a dumbbell in each hand with your palms facing inwards.

○ Lift your right leg behind you and hinge forward from your hips until your right leg and spine are almost parallel to the floor (a).

○ Lift your elbows high, keeping them in by your sides (b).

○ Exhale to press the dumbbells back, straightening and bending your arms eight times (c).

○ Repeat the exercise with your left leg raised.

Quick tip!
Keep your abdominals drawn in, navel to spine. Focus your eyes on one point to aid balance.

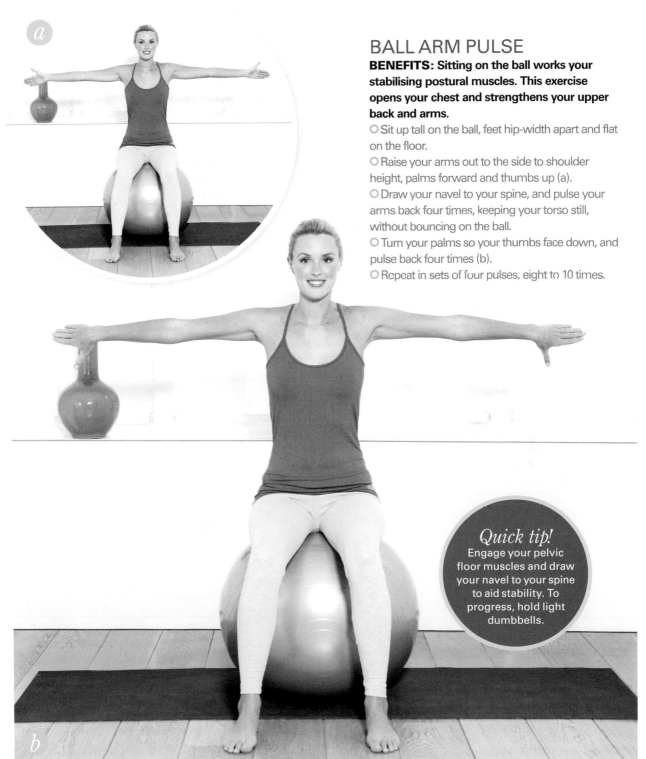

BALL ARM PULSE

BENEFITS: Sitting on the ball works your stabilising postural muscles. This exercise opens your chest and strengthens your upper back and arms.

○ Sit up tall on the ball, feet hip-width apart and flat on the floor.

○ Raise your arms out to the side to shoulder height, palms forward and thumbs up (a).

○ Draw your navel to your spine, and pulse your arms back four times, keeping your torso still, without bouncing on the ball.

○ Turn your palms so your thumbs face down, and pulse back four times (b).

○ Repeat in sets of four pulses, eight to 10 times.

Quick tip!
Engage your pelvic floor muscles and draw your navel to your spine to aid stability. To progress, hold light dumbbells.

PERFECT POSTURE MOVES

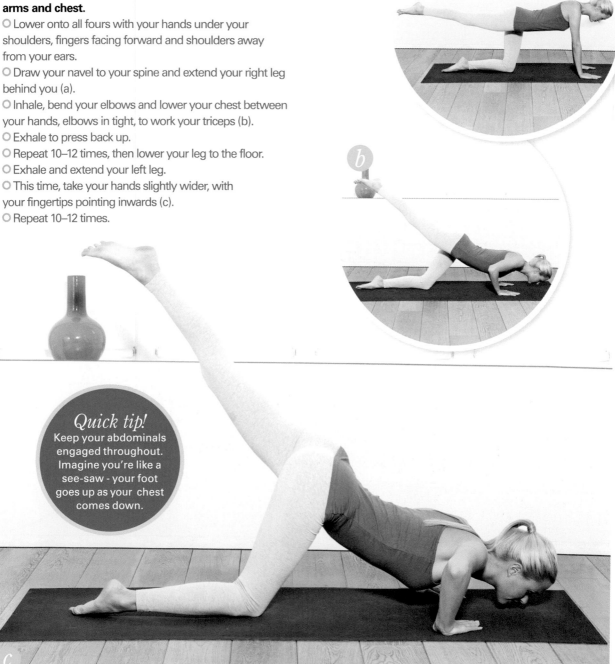

PERFECT POSTURE MOVES

CAT PRESS

BENEFITS: Strengthens your core, bottom, upper arms and chest.

○ Lower onto all fours with your hands under your shoulders, fingers facing forward and shoulders away from your ears.

○ Draw your navel to your spine and extend your right leg behind you (a).

○ Inhale, bend your elbows and lower your chest between your hands, elbows in tight, to work your triceps (b).

○ Exhale to press back up.

○ Repeat 10–12 times, then lower your leg to the floor.

○ Exhale and extend your left leg.

○ This time, take your hands slightly wider, with your fingertips pointing inwards (c).

○ Repeat 10–12 times.

Quick tip!
Keep your abdominals engaged throughout. Imagine you're like a see-saw - your foot goes up as your chest comes down.

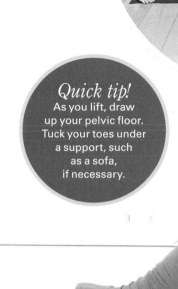

BALL BACK EXTENSION

BENEFITS: Works your core, back and postural muscles.

O Lie on an exercise ball, face down and legs wide for support.

O Place your fingertips under your forehead, palms facing down (a).

O Exhale and raise your head and shoulders off the ball (b).

O Inhale and lower back down.

O Repeat 10–12 times.

Quick tip!
As you lift, draw up your pelvic floor. Tuck your toes under a support, such as a sofa, if necessary.

PERFECT POSTURE CIRCUIT

Good posture is not only instantly slimming, it helps prevent back problems. If your muscles are hunched, your internal organs will also be cramped and unable to function efficiently. For

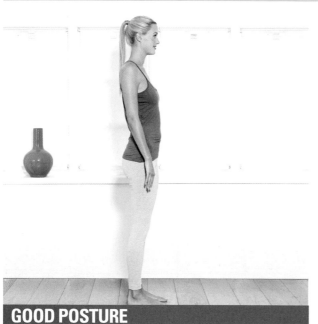

GOOD POSTURE

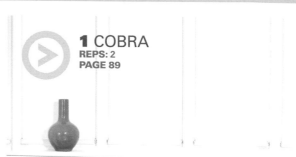

1 COBRA
REPS: 2
PAGE 89

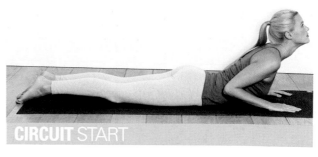

CIRCUIT START

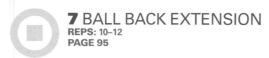

7 BALL BACK EXTENSION
REPS: 10–12
PAGE 95

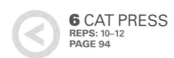

6 CAT PRESS
REPS: 10–12
PAGE 94

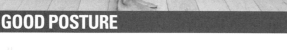

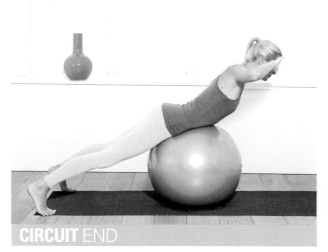

CIRCUIT END

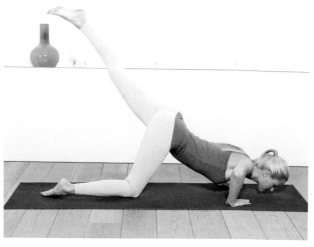

general maintenance and a great workout, repeat one to two times a week. If you know your posture needs some work, add an extra session to your weekly routine.

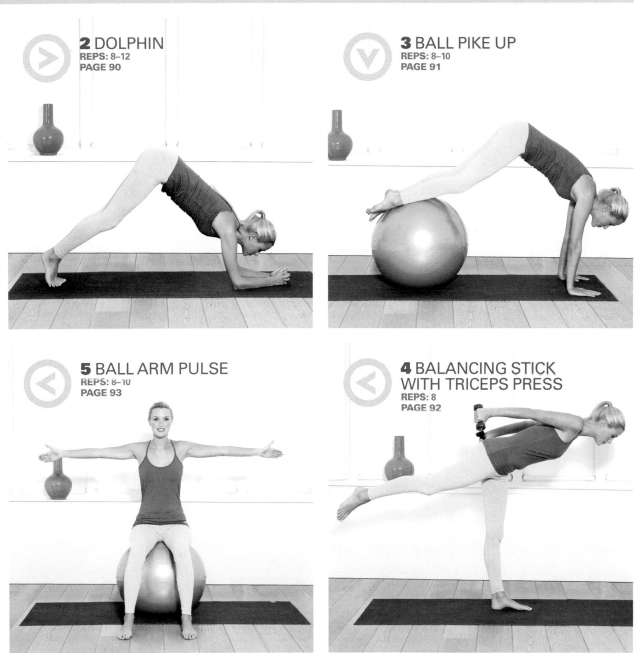

2 DOLPHIN
REPS: 8–12
PAGE 90

3 BALL PIKE UP
REPS: 8–10
PAGE 91

5 BALL ARM PULSE
REPS: 8–10
PAGE 93

4 BALANCING STICK
WITH TRICEPS PRESS
REPS: 8
PAGE 92

PERFECT POSTURE CIRCUIT

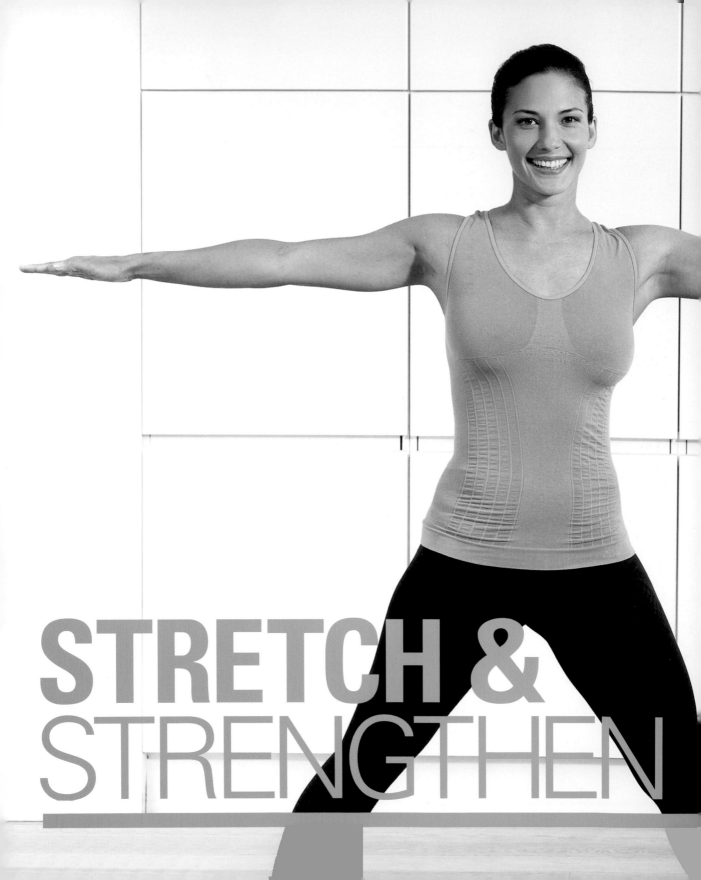

STRETCH &
STRENGTHEN

Get a lean, supple body for life with these easy-flex moves

Flexibility is a vital component of a fit and healthy body. You should always stretch after workouts, but it's also important to devote time to flexibility sessions. Stiff muscles and joints will prevent correct movement and can cause injury and pain, and as yoga teachers will tell you, you're only as young as your spine is flexible!

As you age, it's natural to lose some flexibility – a baby can easily put its foot into its own mouth, but as we age, we only do this metaphorically! If nothing is done to prevent it, many people end up with a stiff and hunched posture in their later years. While you can't hope to keep your body as mobile as a baby's, you can aim to keep your spine and joints flexible and your muscles pliable well into old age.

It's important to take your joints through their full range of movement. Your hip, for example, is a ball and socket joint designed to move back and forth, side to side and in circles. Often, however, it's only used in a backwards and forwards movement, as in sitting, standing, walking or running, for example. But if you don't use it, you lose it!

Yoga is great for opening the hips and keeping the muscles supple, and by adding this routine into your exercise programme at least once a week, you'll help your body stay young and free.

The following moves are all designed to strengthen your body as well as increase flexibility.

EXERCISE ONE

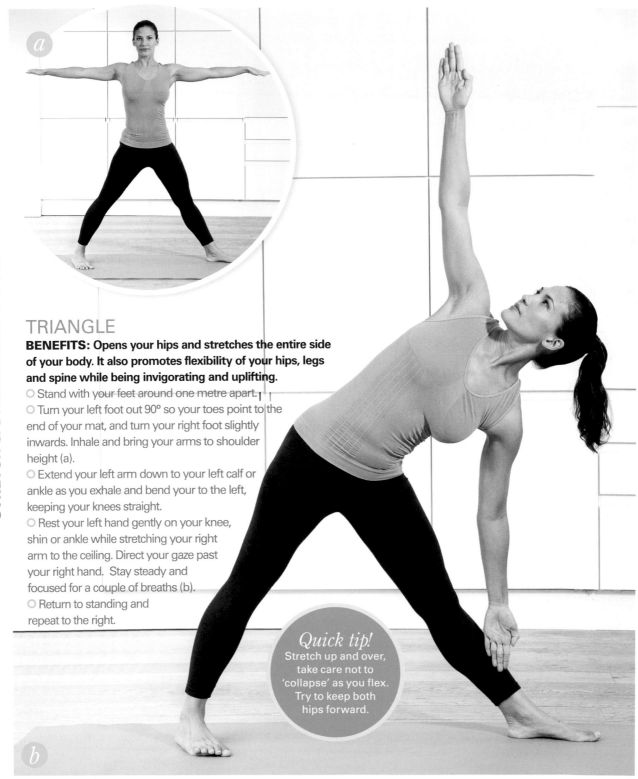

a

STRETCH & STRENGTHEN MOVES

TRIANGLE

BENEFITS: Opens your hips and stretches the entire side of your body. It also promotes flexibility of your hips, legs and spine while being invigorating and uplifting.

○ Stand with your feet around one metre apart.
○ Turn your left foot out 90º so your toes point to the end of your mat, and turn your right foot slightly inwards. Inhale and bring your arms to shoulder height (a).
○ Extend your left arm down to your left calf or ankle as you exhale and bend your to the left, keeping your knees straight.
○ Rest your left hand gently on your knee, shin or ankle while stretching your right arm to the ceiling. Direct your gaze past your right hand. Stay steady and focused for a couple of breaths (b).
○ Return to standing and repeat to the right.

Quick tip!
Stretch up and over, take care not to 'collapse' as you flex. Try to keep both hips forward.

b

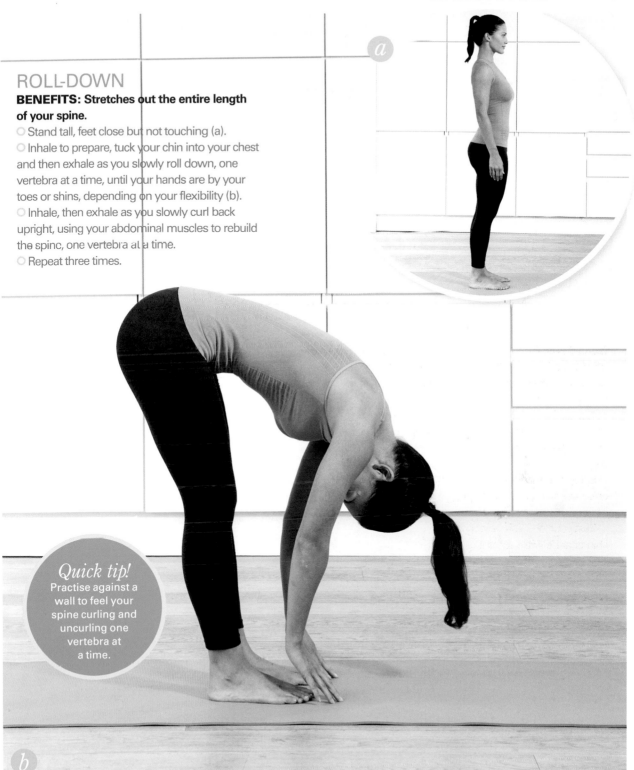

ROLL-DOWN

BENEFITS: Stretches out the entire length of your spine.

○ Stand tall, feet close but not touching (a).

○ Inhale to prepare, tuck your chin into your chest and then exhale as you slowly roll down, one vertebra at a time, until your hands are by your toes or shins, depending on your flexibility (b).

○ Inhale, then exhale as you slowly curl back upright, using your abdominal muscles to rebuild the spine, one vertebra at a time.

○ Repeat three times.

Quick tip!
Practise against a wall to feel your spine curling and uncurling one vertebra at a time.

STRETCH & STRENGTHEN MOVES

STRETCH & STRENGTHEN MOVES

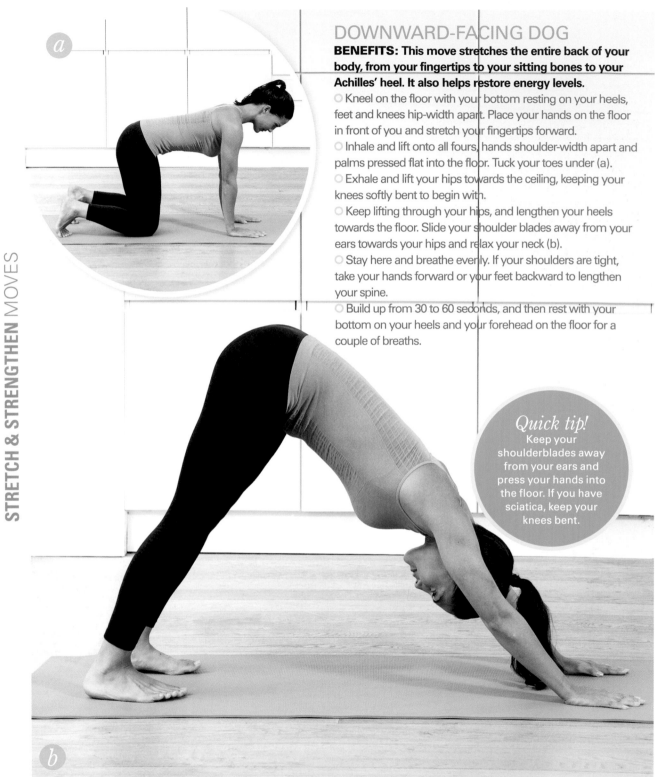

DOWNWARD-FACING DOG

BENEFITS: This move stretches the entire back of your body, from your fingertips to your sitting bones to your Achilles' heel. It also helps restore energy levels.

◯ Kneel on the floor with your bottom resting on your heels, feet and knees hip-width apart. Place your hands on the floor in front of you and stretch your fingertips forward.

◯ Inhale and lift onto all fours, hands shoulder-width apart and palms pressed flat into the floor. Tuck your toes under (a).

◯ Exhale and lift your hips towards the ceiling, keeping your knees softly bent to begin with.

◯ Keep lifting through your hips, and lengthen your heels towards the floor. Slide your shoulder blades away from your ears towards your hips and relax your neck (b).

◯ Stay here and breathe evenly. If your shoulders are tight, take your hands forward or your feet backward to lengthen your spine.

◯ Build up from 30 to 60 seconds, and then rest with your bottom on your heels and your forehead on the floor for a couple of breaths.

Quick tip!
Keep your shoulderblades away from your ears and press your hands into the floor. If you have sciatica, keep your knees bent.

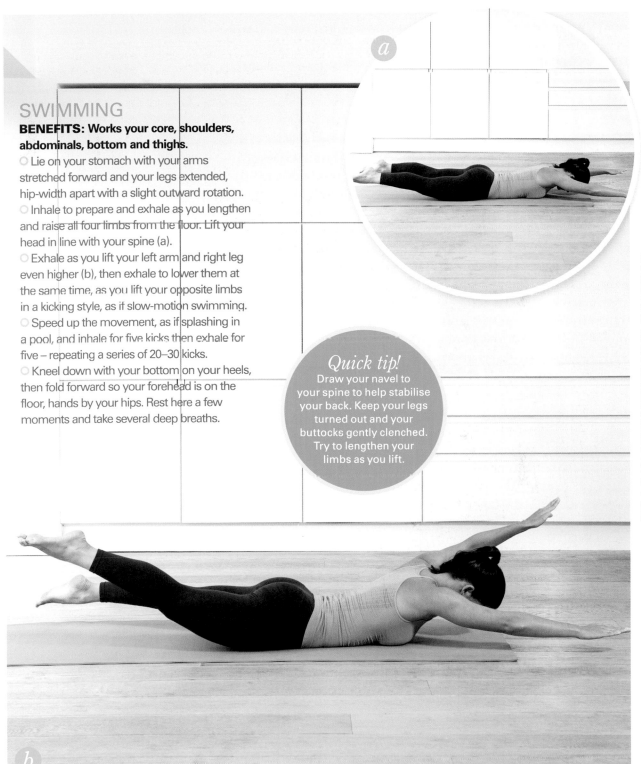

SWIMMING

BENEFITS: Works your core, shoulders, abdominals, bottom and thighs.

○ Lie on your stomach with your arms stretched forward and your legs extended, hip-width apart with a slight outward rotation.

○ Inhale to prepare and exhale as you lengthen and raise all four limbs from the floor. Lift your head in line with your spine (a).

○ Exhale as you lift your left arm and right leg even higher (b), then exhale to lower them at the same time, as you lift your opposite limbs in a kicking style, as if slow-motion swimming.

○ Speed up the movement, as if splashing in a pool, and inhale for five kicks then exhale for five – repeating a series of 20–30 kicks.

○ Kneel down with your bottom on your heels, then fold forward so your forehead is on the floor, hands by your hips. Rest here a few moments and take several deep breaths.

Quick tip!
Draw your navel to your spine to help stabilise your back. Keep your legs turned out and your buttocks gently clenched. Try to lengthen your limbs as you lift.

STRETCH & STRENGTHEN MOVES

STRETCH & STRENGTHEN MOVES

HEEL SQUEEZE PRONE

BENEFITS: Great for strengthening and sculpting your bottom.

○ Lie face down with your forehead supported on the back of your hands.

○ Bend your knees and take them shoulder-width apart, keeping your heels touching.

○ Keep your spine in neutral.

○ Inhale, then exhale and press your heels together, squeezing your bottom tightly for a count of four (pictured). Inhale to release.

○ Repeat eight times.

Quick tip!
Keep your spine neutral throughout and your abdominals drawn in.

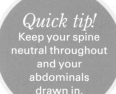

BOW

BENEFITS: This backward bend counteracts a hunched spine, while strengthening your back and aiding digestion.

○ Lie on your stomach with your forehead on the floor. Raise your head, bend your knees and reach back with both hands to grasp your ankles (a).

○ Keeping your arms straight, inhale as you push your feet backwards, lifting your head, shoulders and chest upwards, keeping your gaze down to the floor (b).

○ Hold this position and breathe evenly for three to six breaths.

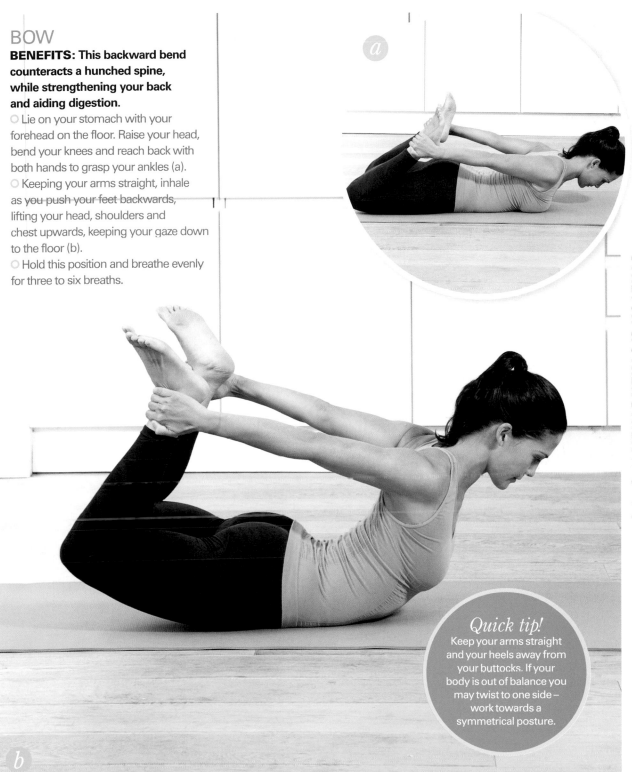

STRETCH & STRENGTHEN MOVES

Quick tip!
Keep your arms straight and your heels away from your buttocks. If your body is out of balance you may twist to one side – work towards a symmetrical posture.

a

SHOULDER BRIDGE

BENEFITS: This beginner's version of the bridge is a gentle inversion, which mobilises your spine, stretches out the front of your hips and strengthens your hamstrings and gluteals.

○ Lie on your back with your arms by your sides, palms facing down. Bend both knees and place your feet flat on the floor, hip-width apart and close to your buttocks (a).

○ Inhale, then exhale as you raise your hips, placing your hands flat on your back for support, with your fingers pointing in towards your spine (b).

○ Keep your hips high, arch your chest upwards and breathe deeply for eight to 10 breaths.

○ Return your hips to the floor, and draw your knees to your chest to counter-stretch your spine.

Quick tip!
Keep your knees hip-width apart, toes pointing forward, feet parallel. Keep your head central and still.

b

SPINAL TWIST

BENEFITS: Stretches and twists your spine, stretches your hips and shoulders, massages your abdominal organs and aids digestive problems. Relaxes and centres.

- Sit on your heels with a straight spine.
- Support your weight with your left hand as you transfer your weight to your left hip. Place your right foot flat on the floor on the outside of your left knee (a).
- Lengthen your spine then twist around to the right, your left elbow on the outside of your right knee. Your right hand is on the floor close to your right hip (b). Hold for a few breaths.
- Repeat on the other side.

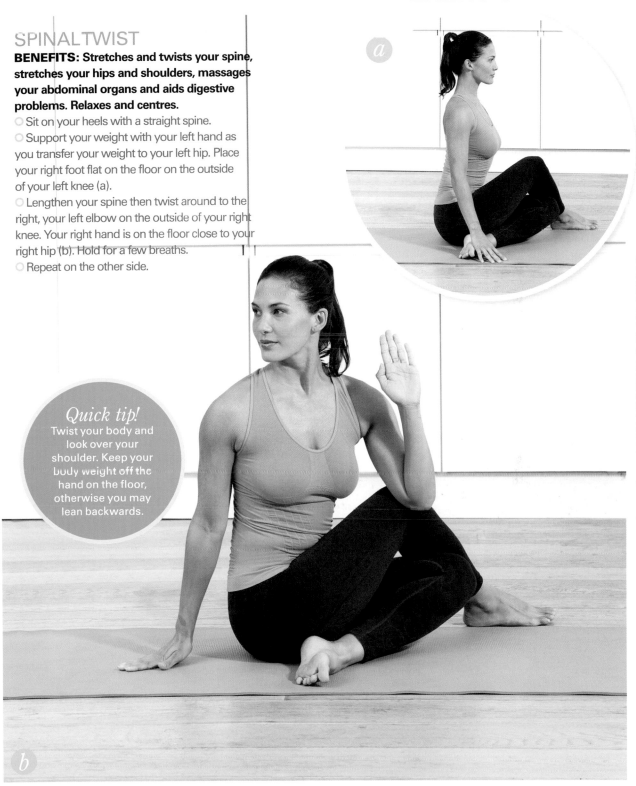

a

b

Quick tip!
Twist your body and look over your shoulder. Keep your body weight off the hand on the floor, otherwise you may lean backwards.

STRETCH & STRENGTHEN MOVES

STRETCH & STRENGTHEN CIRCUIT

Not only will stretching help reduce soreness after exercise, if your body is flexible you'll perform better in your workouts. You'll benefit more from your yoga and Pilates postures, your

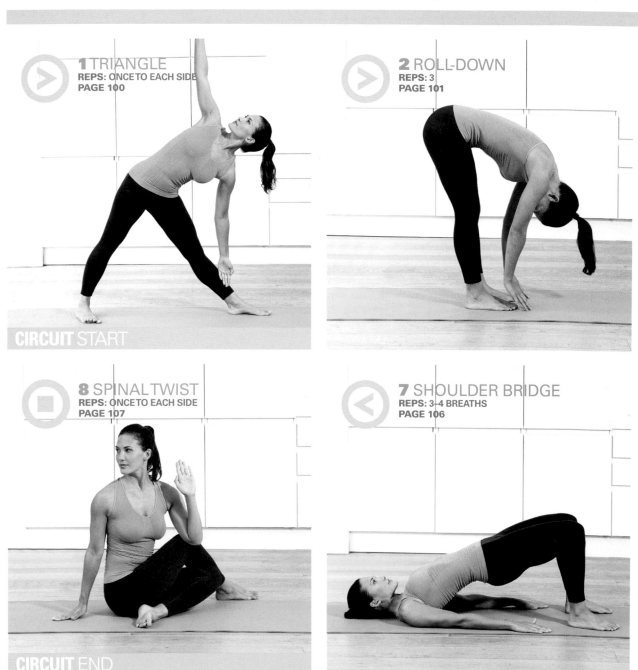

1 TRIANGLE
REPS: ONCE TO EACH SIDE
PAGE 100

CIRCUIT START

2 ROLL-DOWN
REPS: 3
PAGE 101

8 SPINAL TWIST
REPS: ONCE TO EACH SIDE
PAGE 107

CIRCUIT END

7 SHOULDER BRIDGE
REPS: 3–4 BREATHS
PAGE 106

running style will improve and, as your muscles gain strength, you'll be able to sustain your workouts for longer. More muscle tone will give your body better definition too.

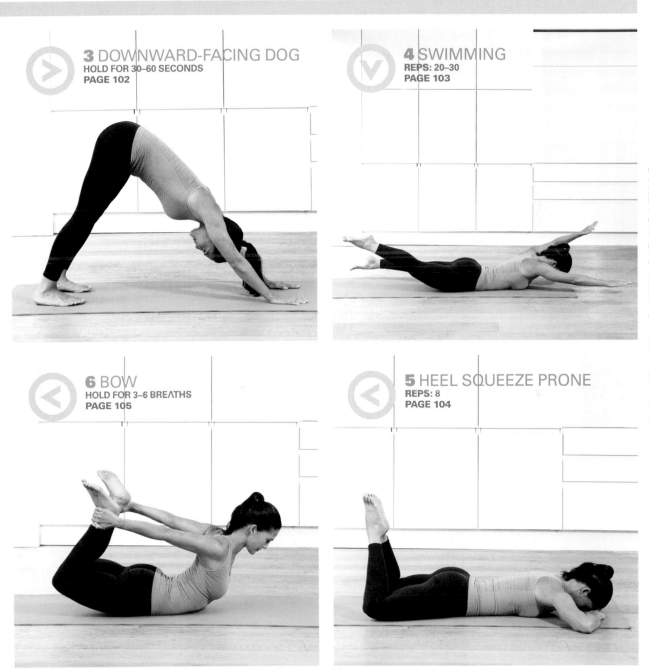

3 DOWNWARD-FACING DOG
HOLD FOR 30–60 SECONDS
PAGE 102

4 SWIMMING
REPS: 20–30
PAGE 103

6 BOW
HOLD FOR 3–6 BREATHS
PAGE 105

5 HEEL SQUEEZE PRONE
REPS: 8
PAGE 104

STRETCH & STRENGTHEN CIRCUIT

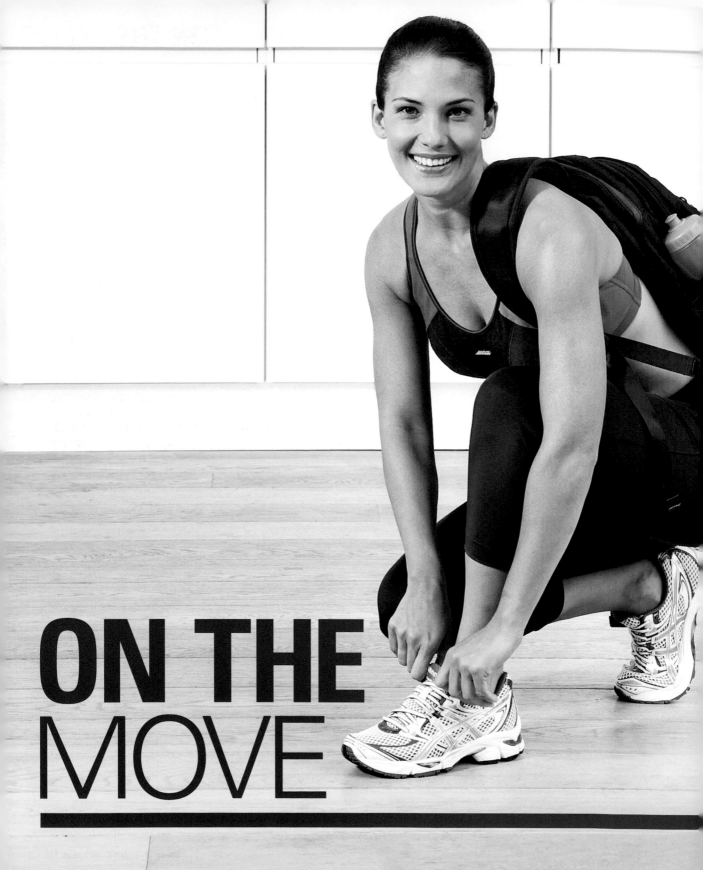

ON THE
MOVE

Stay fit when you're away from home with this do-anywhere circuit

Whether you're travelling for work, **away on holiday or in the office for long hours, you can still get a great all-body workout using nothing but your own body weight and a chair!**

Being away from home frequently can make exercising hard, but this routine will banish that problem so you can maintain your tone and strength no matter where you are.

This programme is based around resistance exercises to strengthen and tone your muscles.

For your cardiovascular workout, if you're staying in a friendly, well-lit neighbourhood, you could go out for a run or walk. This is an ideal way to get to know the vicinity, and can offer you some valuable 'me time' too. If you don't feel comfortable in an unknown area and there are no gym facilities to hand, put on your trainers, turn up the air-conditioning and dance your heart out for 30 minutes. Alternatively, mix up running on the spot, towel jumps (see page 59), skipping with an imaginary rope (it works!) and some good old-fashioned star jumps for half an hour.

If you're away on a beach holiday, use what Mother Nature provides – striding in the surf is a great lower-body toner which also works your cardiovascular system. Running on the sand makes your body work a bit harder than running on pavements so you'll burn more calories.

So, whether you're away for work or pleasure, in a hotel or a youth hostel, the most important thing is you move your body, raise your heart rate and have some fun!

ON THE MOVE MOVES

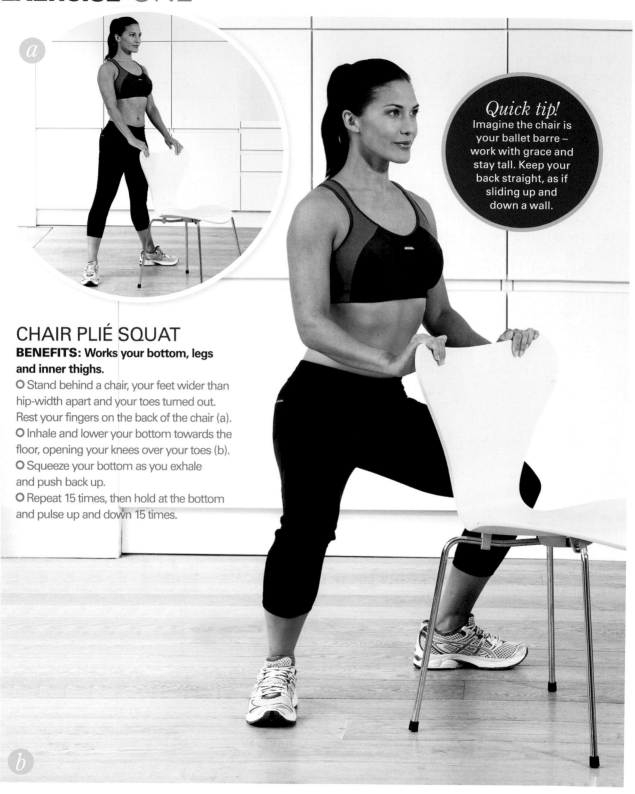

Quick tip!
Imagine the chair is
your ballet barre –
work with grace and
stay tall. Keep your
back straight, as if
sliding up and
down a wall.

CHAIR PLIÉ SQUAT

BENEFITS: Works your bottom, legs and inner thighs.

○ Stand behind a chair, your feet wider than hip-width apart and your toes turned out. Rest your fingers on the back of the chair (a).

○ Inhale and lower your bottom towards the floor, opening your knees over your toes (b).

○ Squeeze your bottom as you exhale and push back up.

○ Repeat 15 times, then hold at the bottom and pulse up and down 15 times.

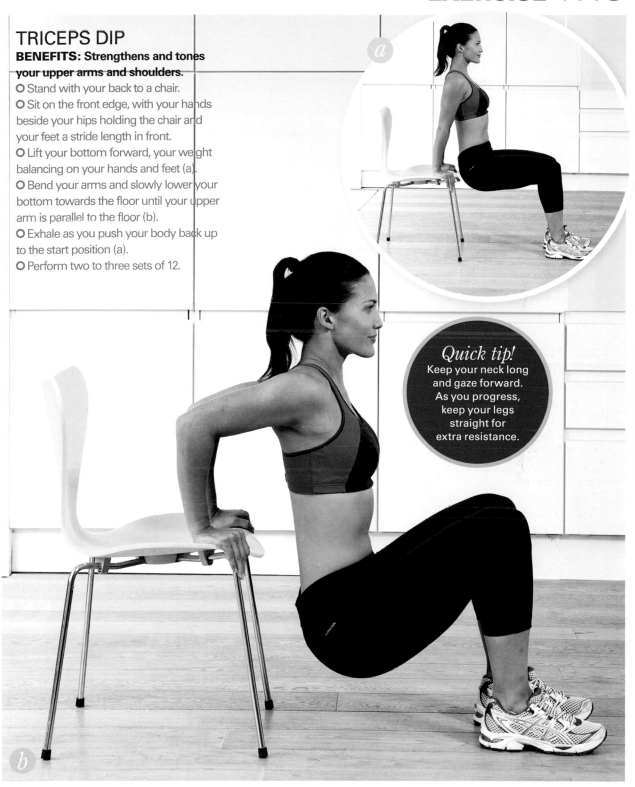

TRICEPS DIP

BENEFITS: Strengthens and tones your upper arms and shoulders.

○ Stand with your back to a chair.

○ Sit on the front edge, with your hands beside your hips holding the chair and your feet a stride length in front.

○ Lift your bottom forward, your weight balancing on your hands and feet (a).

○ Bend your arms and slowly lower your bottom towards the floor until your upper arm is parallel to the floor (b).

○ Exhale as you push your body back up to the start position (a).

○ Perform two to three sets of 12.

Quick tip!
Keep your neck long and gaze forward. As you progress, keep your legs straight for extra resistance.

ON THE MOVE MOVES

EXERCISE THREE

ON THE MOVE MOVES

HIP-RAISER

BENEFITS: This is a great exercise to define and tone your bottom and the backs of your thighs.

○ Lie on your back with your calves on top of a chair, hands by your sides, palms facing down (a).

○ Exhale, squeeze your bottom and lift your hips in the air (b).

○ Inhale as you lower half-way back down, then exhale and continue smoothly into the next lift.

○ Perform two to three sets of 12 reps.

○ As you advance, try single leg reps – as above, but with one foot on the chair, the other leg extended upward (c).

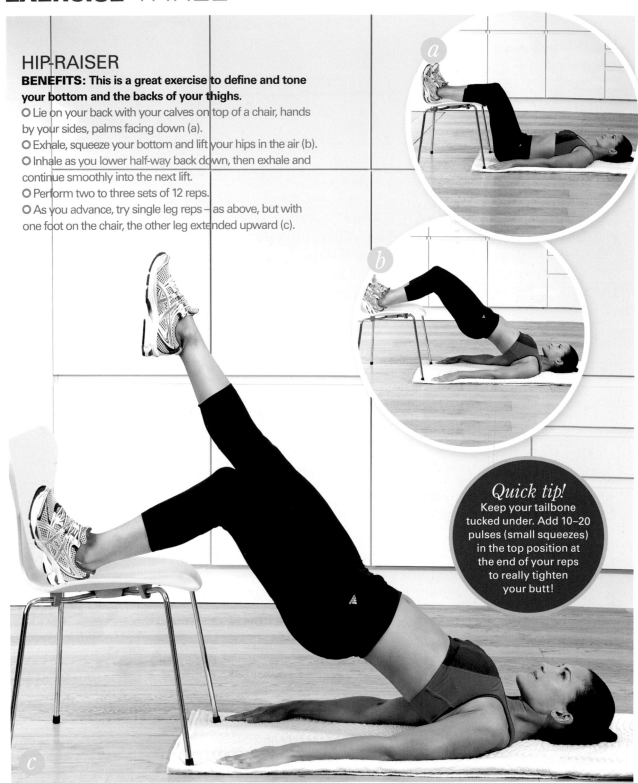

Quick tip!
Keep your tailbone tucked under. Add 10–20 pulses (small squeezes) in the top position at the end of your reps to really tighten your butt!

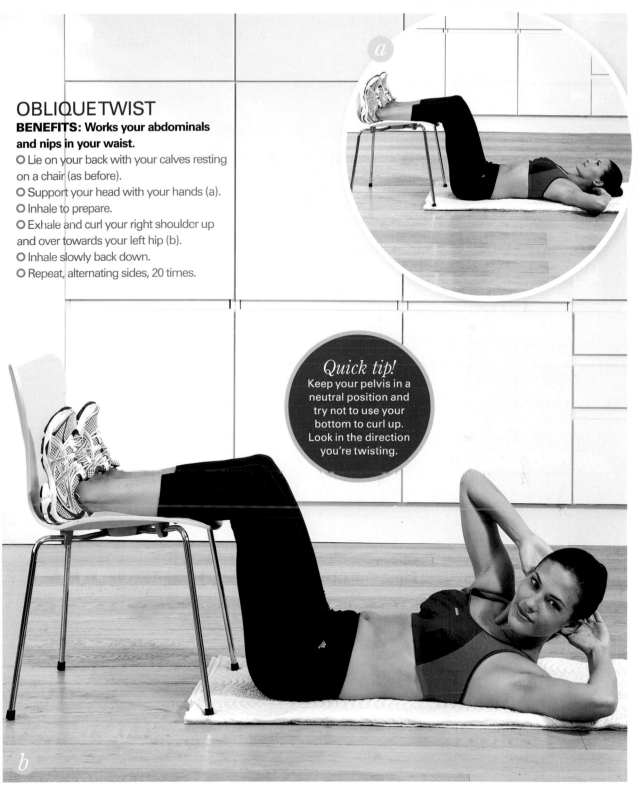

OBLIQUE TWIST

BENEFITS: Works your abdominals and nips in your waist.

○ Lie on your back with your calves resting on a chair (as before).
○ Support your head with your hands (a).
○ Inhale to prepare.
○ Exhale and curl your right shoulder up and over towards your left hip (b).
○ Inhale slowly back down.
○ Repeat, alternating sides, 20 times.

Quick tip!
Keep your pelvis in a neutral position and try not to use your bottom to curl up. Look in the direction you're twisting.

ON THE MOVE MOVES

BUM LIFTER

BENEFITS: Lifts and tones your bottom.

○ Stand behind a chair, holding the backrest for support, arms slightly bent.

○ Raise your right leg straight behind you (a).

○ Lift and lower your leg 10 times.

○ Next, circle your raised leg 10 times clockwise and 10 times anti-clockwise.

○ Finally, look towards your right leg, knee lifted high and straighten and bend it 10 times (b).

○ Repeat the series on the other leg.

Quick tip!
Keep your abdominals drawn in and try not to arch your back as you lift your leg.

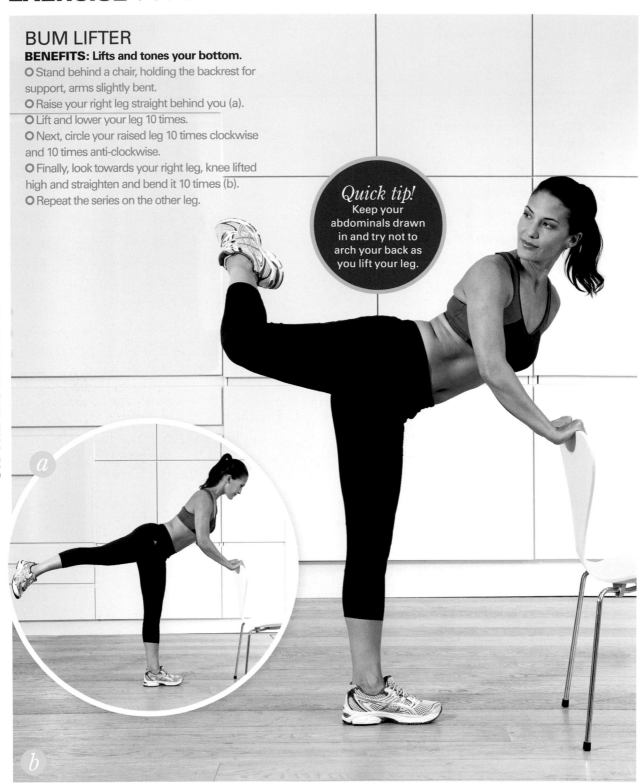

a

b

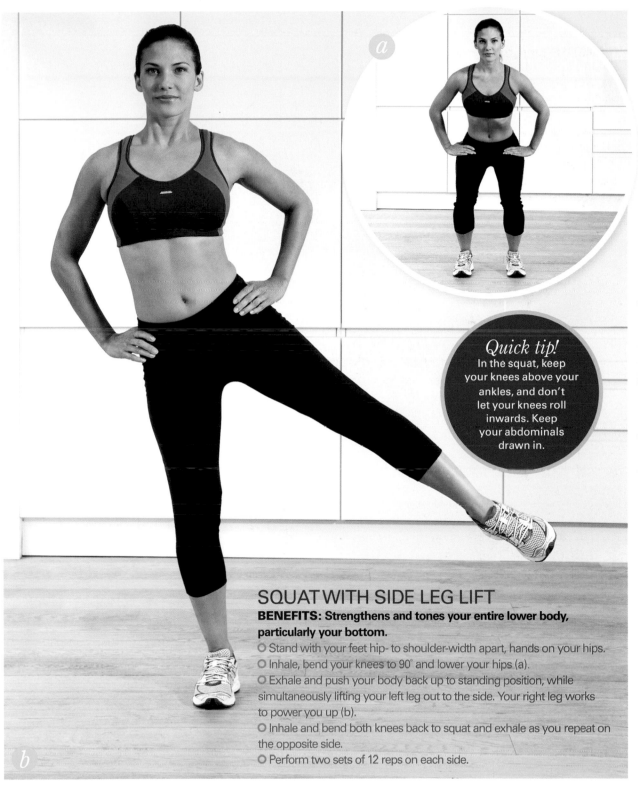

a

b

Quick tip!
In the squat, keep your knees above your ankles, and don't let your knees roll inwards. Keep your abdominals drawn in.

SQUAT WITH SIDE LEG LIFT
BENEFITS: Strengthens and tones your entire lower body, particularly your bottom.

○ Stand with your feet hip- to shoulder-width apart, hands on your hips.

○ Inhale, bend your knees to 90° and lower your hips (a).

○ Exhale and push your body back up to standing position, while simultaneously lifting your left leg out to the side. Your right leg works to power you up (b).

○ Inhale and bend both knees back to squat and exhale as you repeat on the opposite side.

○ Perform two sets of 12 reps on each side.

ON THE MOVE MOVES

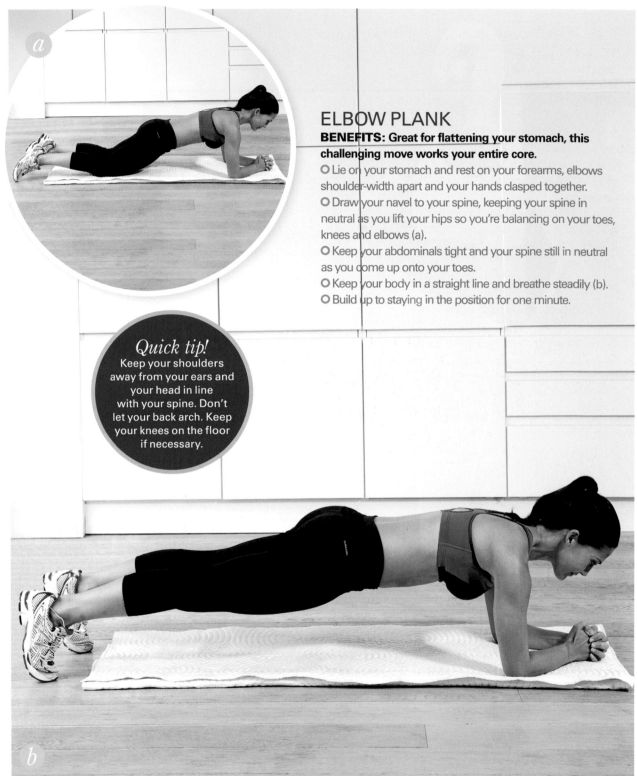

ELBOW PLANK

BENEFITS: Great for flattening your stomach, this challenging move works your entire core.

○ Lie on your stomach and rest on your forearms, elbows shoulder-width apart and your hands clasped together.

○ Draw your navel to your spine, keeping your spine in neutral as you lift your hips so you're balancing on your toes, knees and elbows (a).

○ Keep your abdominals tight and your spine still in neutral as you come up onto your toes.

○ Keep your body in a straight line and breathe steadily (b).

○ Build up to staying in the position for one minute.

Quick tip!
Keep your shoulders away from your ears and your head in line with your spine. Don't let your back arch. Keep your knees on the floor if necessary.

PRESS-UP

**BENEFITS: A challenging old favourite!
Targets your upper body – particularly
your chest and triceps.**

○ Place your hands under your shoulders
and your legs out straight with your weight
on your toes (a). If this is too challenging,
rest on your knees (b).

○ Keep your back straight and inhale as
you lower your chest towards the floor,
bending your elbows (c).

○ Exhale as you press back up to the
start position (a).

○ Build up to three sets of 12 reps.

Quick tip!
Keep your abdominals
and bottom tight.
Placing your hands
wider works your chest
more, placing them
closer together works
your triceps more.

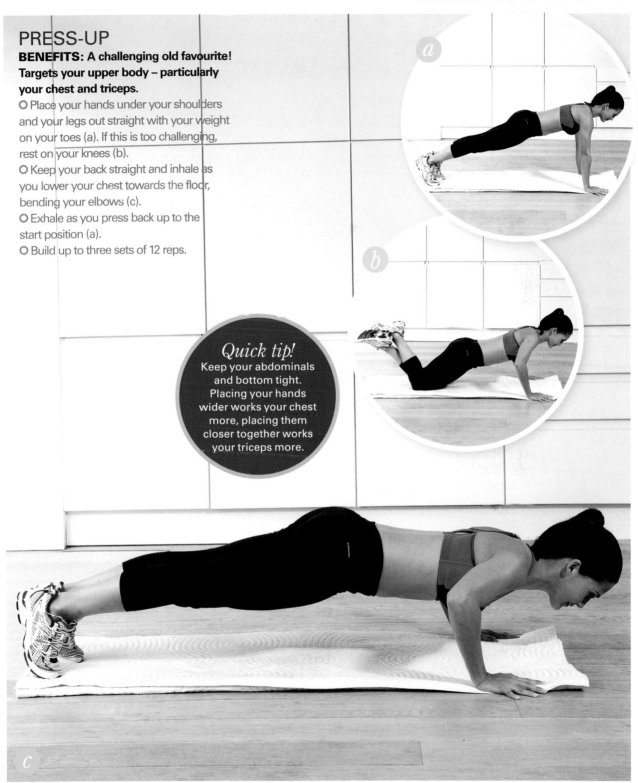

ON THE MOVE MOVES

ON THE MOVE CIRCUIT

If you're staying in a hotel and the floor is hard, use a folded blanket to protect your spine when doing moves that involve lying on your back. Make use of furniture in your room, or

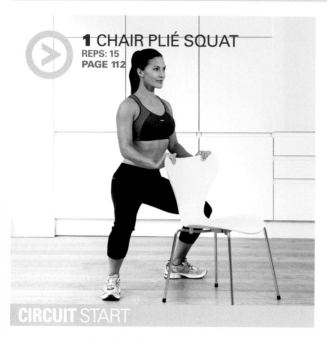

1 CHAIR PLIÉ SQUAT
REPS: 15
PAGE 112

CIRCUIT START

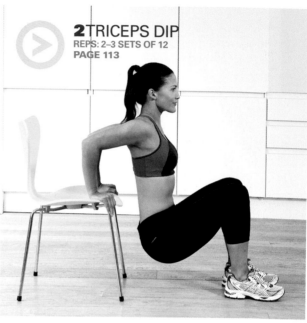

2 TRICEPS DIP
REPS: 2–3 SETS OF 12
PAGE 113

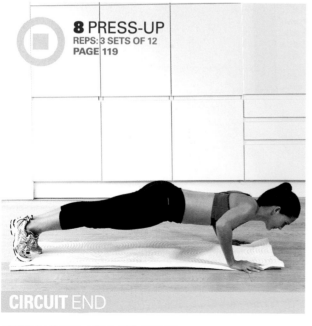

8 PRESS-UP
REPS: 3 SETS OF 12
PAGE 119

CIRCUIT END

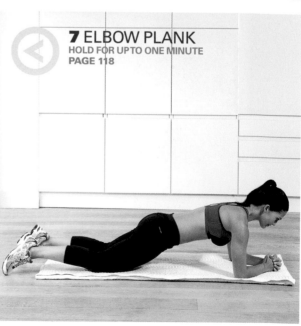

7 ELBOW PLANK
HOLD FOR UP TO ONE MINUTE
PAGE 118

if there's nothing suitable, ask at reception for a hard chair you can borrow for your stay. If you don't have time to complete the circuit in one go, break it up into shorter sections.

3 HIP-RAISER
REPS: 2–3 SETS OF 12
PAGE 114

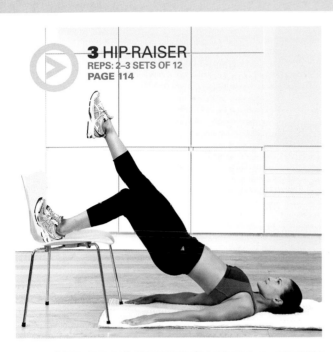

4 OBLIQUE TWIST
REPS: 20 ON EACH SIDE
PAGE 115

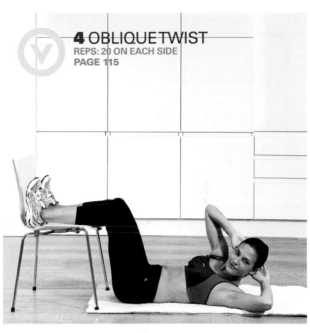

6 SQUAT WITH SIDE
LEG LIFT
REPS: 2 SETS OF 12 ON EACH SIDE
PAGE 117

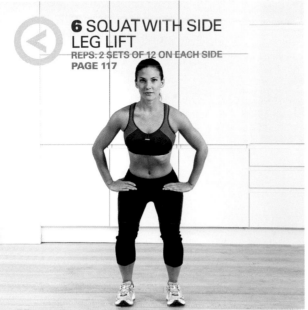

5 BUM LIFTER
REPS: 4 SETS OF 10 ON EACH SIDE
PAGE 116

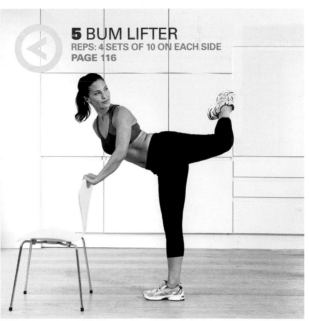

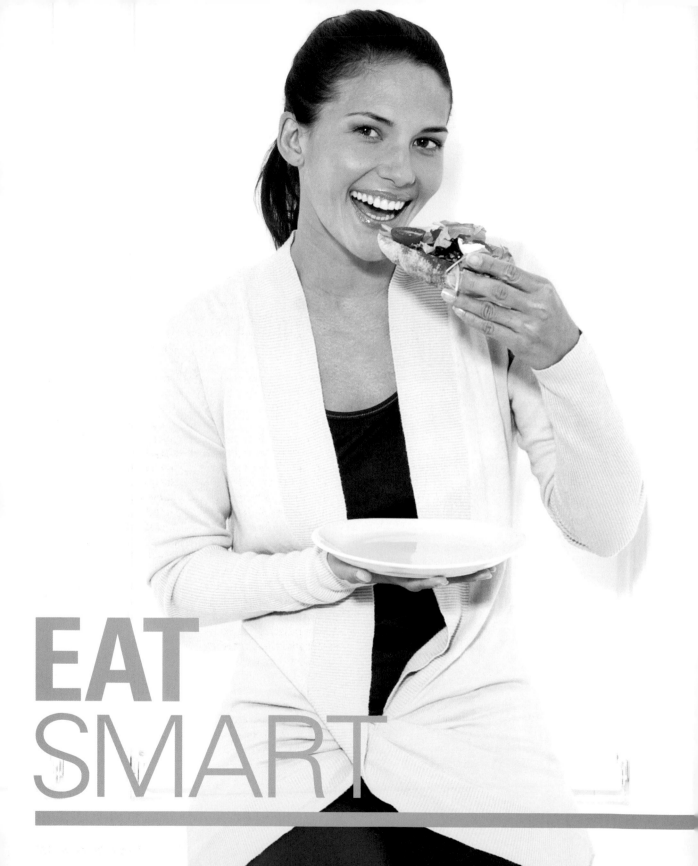

EAT
SMART

Get your eating habits right and you can boost the benefits of your workouts even further

Now you have your exercise routine in place, it's time to think about your diet.

Whether you want to lose pounds or simply maintain a good figure, your diet plays a crucial role. Eating well is also vital to help you get the most from your exercise routine.

When it comes to fuelling workouts, unless you're planning a strenuous challenge, such as running a marathon, you should be able to get the nutrients you need from a normal healthy diet. But there are some important guidelines to consider.

Your muscles use both carbohydrate and protein for fuel, so don't skimp on either of these.

Getting a sufficient intake of vitamins and minerals is also essential for your training. Low levels of calcium and magnesium can lead to muscle cramps, for instance, while adequate iron stores reduce the risk of exercise-induced anaemia. And what you eat also plays a part in helping your muscles recover after a hard workout.

If you're aiming to lose weight, start with a food diary. Make a note of what you eat over two-weeks, along with how you felt before and after eating (were you really hungry, or was it stress that made you succumb to that blueberry muffin?). This can help you understand what triggers your cravings, and help you come up with alternative strategies for successfully managing apparent hunger pangs.

Over the next few pages you'll find out how best to eat to ensure you're full of energy for training, minimise muscle soreness after, and maintain a healthy weight.

EAT FOR A
BETTER BODY

When you're aiming to streamline, tone and strengthen your body, it's not just the exercise side of the equation that matters. The food you eat is important too – and it's not just about cutting down on calories or limiting your fat intake.

What you mustn't do is subject yourself to restrictive or faddy eating plans that leave you with barely enough energy to flick through the TV channels at the end of the day, let alone go out for a run.

The diet that works best will taste good and won't leave you psychologically or physically deprived; it's one that's healthy, but not so strict you can't imagine happily following it as a long-term lifestyle choice.

The dietary guidelines below – based on the latest scientific evidence – are eminently 'do-able' but will give peak results for your body when teamed with exercise.

WHAT TO DO

○ At lunch and dinner, eat approximately equal quantities of low-fat, unprocessed protein (lean meat and poultry, fish, beans or pulses), slow-releasing (low-GI) carbohydrates (wholegrain pasta, rice or sweet potatoes) and fruit and veg.

○ For breakfast (the time and content can be flexible according to when you decide to work out), go for protein and/or low-GI carbohydrate combinations, such as egg on toast, muesli and yoghurt or porridge with milk.

○ Eat a couple of low-fat dairy portions (yoghurt, skimmed milk) each day, which could feature in meals or as snacks. Dairy products enhance fat-loss and provide bone-building calcium and other essential nutrients.

○ Snacks are fine in moderation and can help keep your hunger under control. But factor them into your overall daily calorie allowance and remember to snack smart, as, in many cases, your snack will also be a pre- or post-workout refuelling opportunity.

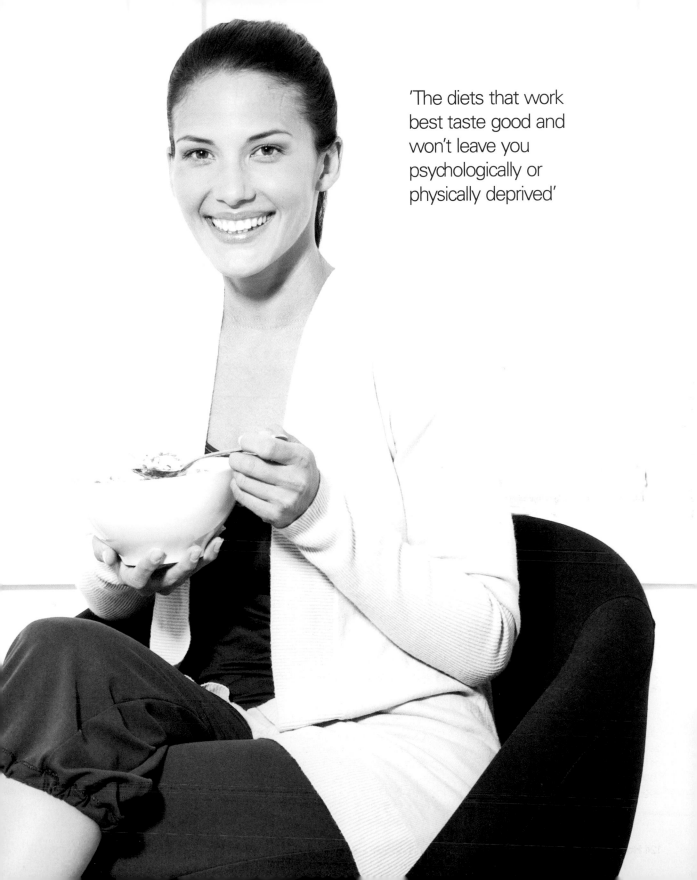

'The diets that work best taste good and won't leave you psychologically or physically deprived'

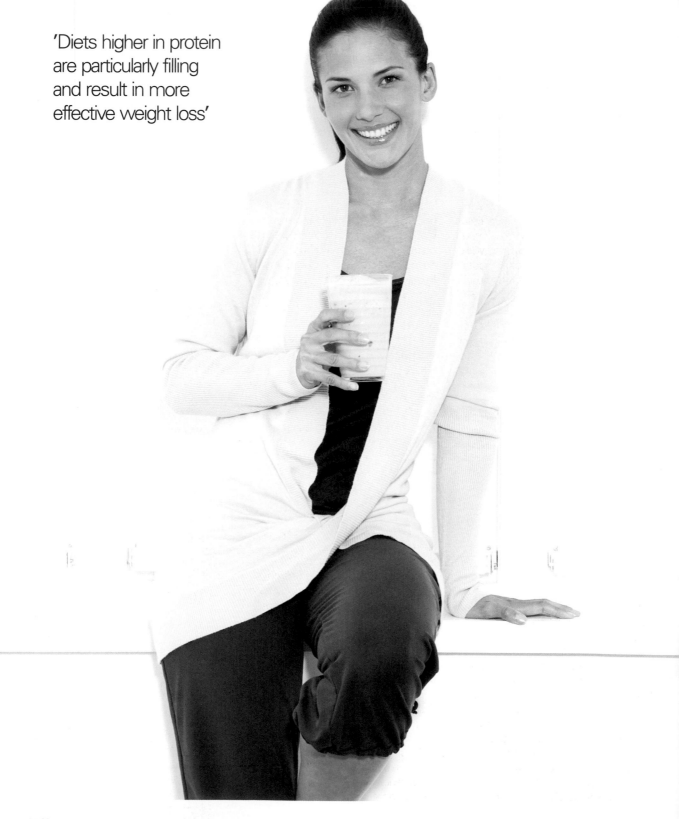

'Diets higher in protein are particularly filling and result in more effective weight loss'

Q: What type of diet should I follow?

If toning up and slimming down is your focus, you need a balanced diet that provides plenty of protein.

According to scientists at the Rowett Institute of Nutrition and Health in Aberdeen, diets higher in protein (lean meat, poultry and fish) are particularly filling and result in more effective weight loss. Protein is also important for the repair and renewal of lean tissue, so it's a vital dietary component if you regularly challenge your muscles with resistance or cardiovascular workouts.

How exactly protein makes you less hungry isn't yet known, but it's possible it slows food transit through the gut or stimulates gut hormones, which promote the feeling of fullness.

High-protein diets may smack of Atkins-style carbohydrate deprivation, but this is only the case if you follow extreme versions. All we're talking about for the purposes of your streamlined, fitter body is a slightly enhanced protein intake – 30 per cent of your calorie intake per meal instead of the 15–20 per cent that's traditionally recommended. You'll still eat good amounts of energy-giving carbohydrates, along with your five-a-day quota of fruit and vegetables.

Q: How many calories a day do I need?

To lose weight at a healthy rate of half a kilo a week, you'll need to create a calorie deficit of 500 a day – which can come from a combination of reducing your normal food intake and expending extra calories by increasing the amount you exercise. Most averagely-active women (for example, those following the workouts in this book) will lose weight at a healthy rate if they eat 1,500 calories a day. If you're averagely-active, you'll maintain your current weight on an intake

of 1,750–2,000 calories a day.

Don't go below 1,200–1,400 calories a day when you're exercising, or you won't have energy to work out and you could end up missing out on essential vitamins and minerals.

Q: When's the best time to eat before exercise?

You'll need to leave at least three hours after a big meal before you work out, but you shouldn't exercise on an empty stomach either. Ideally, have a small meal (for example, a light lunch) or snack containing slow- to medium-releasing carbohydrates and perhaps some protein one to two hours before your workout.

Plan to have a pre-exercise snack if you need to – a banana, or wholegrain mini pitta with a tablespoon of reduced-fat houmous will only supply around 100 calories and are ideal sources of energy. If you're exercising first thing in the morning, have a small snack 40 minutes before your workout and save your breakfast for afterwards.

Q: What should I eat after exercise?

This is a crucial time to eat, as, to maximise recovery, you need to refuel within two hours with carbohydrate and protein (which, research shows, helps carbohydrate storage. If you're not eating a meal within that time, have a snack instead. Post-exercise, your carbohydrates should have a higher GI, so this is one time you could go for white bread and sugary foods.

Some ideal post-training snacks that combine protein and carbohydrates include:

○ 20–30g of nuts and a banana.
○ A boiled egg or chicken sandwich (no spread and, ideally, the white of the egg only for protein without fat).

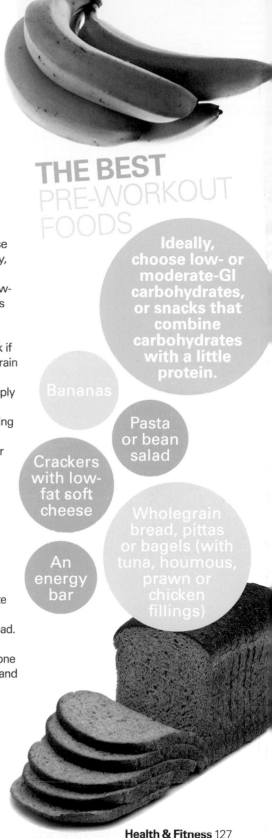

THE BEST PRE-WORKOUT FOODS

Ideally, choose low- or moderate-GI carbohydrates, or snacks that combine carbohydrates with a little protein.

Bananas

Pasta or bean salad

Crackers with low-fat soft cheese

An energy bar

Wholegrain bread, pittas or bagels (with tuna, houmous, prawn or chicken fillings)

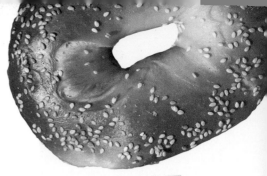

THE BEST RECOVERY FOODS

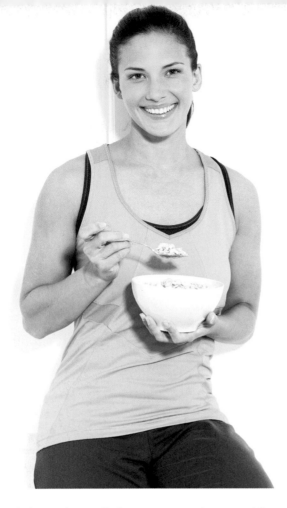

Ideally, choose faster-releasing carbohydrates, but team them with some protein.

White bread or a bagel, with tuna or chicken.

A couple of fish fingers (with a splodge of ketchup).

A banana or handful of jelly beans, followed by a handful of nuts or chunk of reduced-fat Cheddar.

Recovery/protein bars (look at the label and aim to get twice as much carbohydrate as protein).

○ A protein bar and a small glass of fruit juice.

Q: What should I drink?

Eight glasses of water a day is the much-quoted ideal and it's a useful guideline to ensure you're hydrated before exercise. You don't need to stick to it religiously though, nor does everything you drink need to be plain water – tea, coffee, juice, soft drinks and milk count too.

During exercise itself, the range of fluid intake most people need to perform well is between 400 and 1,000ml per hour, depending on the conditions and your activity level.

Water is fine if you plan to exercise for less than an hour and aren't sweating heavily. And if you're only working out for half an hour or so, you can just drink at the end of your workout, providing you made sure you were well hydrated beforehand. If you plan to exercise for longer periods of time, are sweating a lot or just find water unpalatable, an isotonic sports drink can be good for speeding fluid and energy back into the body and replacing lost sodium and potassium.

Q: Do I need sports supplements?

If you're doing only moderate levels of activity, such as the workouts in this book, a healthy balanced diet should give you all the nutrients you need to fuel your workouts and stay healthy. However, isotonic sports drinks and recovery bars can be useful sometimes, especially if you're eating on the go.

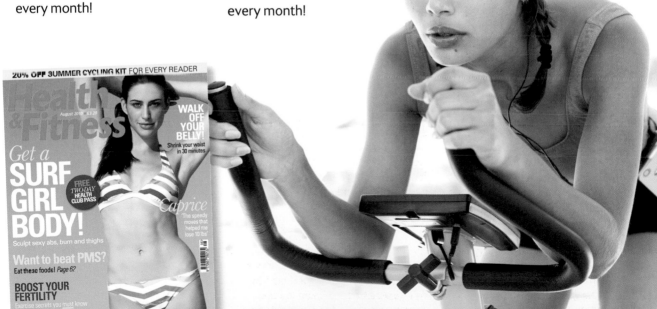

ALL ABOUT YOU

Track your progress by recording your results here!

Record four key areas of your fitness – flexibility, body shape, aerobic capacity and strength in the chart below. Repeat the measurements every four weeks.

Your flexibility

To test your flexibility, sit on the floor with your spine straight and legs extended. Bend from the hips and see how far you can extend your fingers in front of you. See www.topendsports.com/testing/tests/home-sit-and-reach.htm. Make a note of the result.

Your body shape

Measure your bust (just above the nipple line), your waist (around your belly button), your thigh (about a quarter of the way down) and your bottom (at its widest point). Note the results.

Your aerobic fitness

Measure your resting heart rate by feeling your pulse on your wrist after sitting down for a few minutes (count for six seconds then multiply by 10). Then do a step test: step up and down on a stair or low bench, maintaining a steady rhythm for three minutes. Record your heart rate again one minute after. As the weeks progress this figure will decrease and your heart will return more quickly to its resting rate.

Your strength

Count how many press-ups you can complete with good form in a minute. If you're a complete beginner, perform them with your knees on the mat until you're stronger. Also do minute tests for sit-ups and squats.

PROGRESS CHART

	WEEK 1	WEEK 4	WEEK 8	WEEK 12
FLEXIBILITY				
BUST				
WAIST				
THIGHS				
BOTTOM				
RESTING PULSE				
RECOVERING PULSE				
STEP TEST				
PRESS-UP				
SIT-UP				
SQUAT				